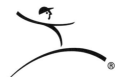

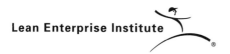

ISBN 978-1-934109-27-4
Design by Off-Piste Design
August 2012

Lean Enterprise Institute, Inc.
215 First Street, Suite 300
Cambridge, MA, 02142 USA
(t) 617-871-2900 • (f) 617-871-2999 • lean.org

On the Mend

Revolutionizing Healthcare
to Save Lives and Transform
the Industry

by John Toussaint, MD
and Roger A. Gerard, PhD

with Emily Adams

Foreword
from the Publisher

Across the world for nearly a century, managers and front-line workers have been steadily learning about the power of rigorous processes to create more value for customers with less waste of every sort—time, defects, human effort, capital investment, injuries. The most accomplished practitioner of these methods through much of the past 60 years has been the Toyota company, but recently many organizations in a wide range of industries far beyond manufacturing have applied rigorous process management—often called lean thinking—to their core activities. When customer value is clearly understood and managers and employees at every level are creatively engaged in dramatically improving traditional processes, the results are invariably highly positive.

Curiously healthcare, with its strong base in the scientific method of rigorous experiments, was largely absent from this movement until recently. Seemingly the steady advance in medical knowledge, including celebrated "miracle cures" like organ transplants and stents to open heart arteries, obscured the fact that the healthcare actually being delivered to the average patient was costly and of low quality in comparison with the results being achieved in many other industries.

In the mid-1990s a few healthcare providers began to experiment with improving their delivery processes. But it took time to modify the improvement tools developed in very different contexts for successful use in healthcare. And there seemed to be little demand for these tools, even once fully proved, as long as the healthcare community believed that traditional management practices and delivery methods were adequate.

But now everything has changed dramatically. As health insurance is extended to millions of additional Americans while the baby-boom generation begins to make significant demands on medical care and government finances grow ever more perilous, the prevailing attitude about traditional methods of healthcare delivery has been radically transformed. Indeed, the one—the only?—thing that all observers of American healthcare can agree on today is that the way we have done things in the past cannot be the way we do things in the future. In consequence, there is suddenly a widespread demand for a simple, actionable approach to creating lean healthcare delivery systems with much lower costs and much better quality. Describing this concept, demonstrating its power to improve results, and explaining how to deploy it is the objective of this book.

Even as we at the Lean Enterprise Institute waited for the healthcare community to embrace lean thinking, we were searching for the leader or leaders best equipped to deliver the message when the time was right. We observed many experimenters in many medical systems with startling results in isolated applications. But we were seeking someone who had brought all of the techniques of lean healthcare together in a complete system—primary care, hospitals, and developed supporting management systems that engaged every employee. We were therefore delighted when we encountered John Toussaint, MD, and his collaborator Roger Gerard, PhD, just as they were completing a decade-long effort to introduce lean healthcare as leaders of the ThedaCare medical system in Wisconsin.

As a doctor, medical director, and then CEO, John Toussaint has taken a hands-on role in pioneering a rigorous approach to quality while slashing waste and cost and improving patient experience across the enterprise. Roger Gerard, as ThedaCare's expert in organizational development and learning, has given hard thought to the change management process and the new leadership behaviors needed to engage doctors, nurses, support staff, and managers in a better approach to providing care while improving their work experience. Together they possess a unique insight on the challenges and rewards of lean healthcare and the book in your hands is the distillation of what they have learned.

One of the key points of this volume is that to embrace lean healthcare you—particularly if you are the senior leader—must *do* lean healthcare by going to the gemba, the place near the bedside where value is actually created for the patient. You need to involve yourself directly in process improvements and learn to see both waste and value. The improvement initiatives described in the pages ahead do not require your direct and undivided participation because of your technical knowledge or authority. Indeed, both may get in the way. Rather you need to apply your hands directly to resolving the problems you will find as part of an improvement team of doctors, nurses, support staff, line managers, and patients because this is how you will change your own thinking about waste, value, and leadership in healthcare.

This prospect is frightening at first for most leaders because they have been trained in a management model where the senior leader (particularly when a doctor) should know all the answers. In fact, lean leaders can only know how to ask the right questions in a collaborative spirit. Your leadership team will probably need help in transitioning from one way of leading to the other. We have therefore helped create the Healthcare Value Network across North America. It is open to any healthcare provider with a leadership that is truly committed to transforming their entire enterprise through hands-on learning and sharing gemba experiences. The work of the Network is described in the End Note. We hope you will consider joining.

Speaking both as the publisher and as a 30-year participant in efforts to introduce lean thinking in a wide range of industries, let me express my hope that you will find *On the Mend* helpful in focusing your own efforts. And let me express the additional hope that you will share your experiences with the multitude of other organizations now embarking on lean healthcare. But let me also urge you to keep clearly in mind your training as medical scientists. Lean transformation is all about Dr. Deming's Plan Do Study Act (PDSA), otherwise known as the scientific method. There is no simple formula to copy and no quick path to success. Instead you must perform your own experiments— tailored to the mission and circumstances of your organization. And then you must honestly study the results and act on your findings, including sharing them with the healthcare community.

The new temptation in these difficult times for healthcare is not to cling to the past. Instead it is to seek quick, painless miracle cures, and someone will always be offering these. But there are no miracle cures, not even "lean" ones, for poorly designed processes, outmoded leadership styles, and unengaged employees. There are only continuous experiments, conducted honestly by leaders with courage, an open mind, and a collaborative spirit, as the healthcare community commences a long journey in pursuit of lean healthcare.

James P. Womack
Founder and Chairman
Lean Enterprise Institute
Cambridge, MA
June 2010

Contents

To my daughter Elizabeth and my son Ted who continue to inspire me with their passion and energy to make the world a better place; and to my wife Susan who has given unending support and love in so many difficult times—*thank you.*

– John

To my wife, Debra; my son, Avery; my daughters, Meghan, Laura, and Erin, and their spouses and children; and especially to my father, Gerald Gerard (deceased), who was a lifetime hero and role model of everything a father and a man should be. Thanks, Dad, for all you've given.

– Roger

Inside
the Black Box

Every time you walk into a hospital or clinic in the United States, you take your life in your hands. Whatever your condition, you will probably be cared for by people who are overworked and hobbled by wasteful systems. With 15 million incidents of medical harm[1] in the United States every year, such as drug errors, wrong-site surgeries, and infection, there is a good chance you will be hurt in this interaction. Medical professionals like us are horrified every time we cause harm, but even the best intentions do not change facts.

Meanwhile, government policy makers argue about the healthcare crisis and focus almost exclusively on money—who pays, how much, and from what budget. From the sidelines, we have been repeatedly struck by how little the players seem to know about how healthcare is actually provided. It is as if they are talking about a black box they have never cracked open to investigate, so they can only talk about

---

1. The Institute for Healthcare Improvement, http://www.ihi.org/IHI/Programs/Campaign

the environment surrounding the box—about changing payment systems to providers, insurance coverage for patients, and reporting requirements for healthcare organizations. These prescriptions are based on one abstract theory or another with no real insight into why healthcare costs so much. With few exceptions, the debaters assume that healthcare costs are fixed, that America's proud history of medical care and innovation comes with a staggering bill.

We know different.

Governments can tweak payment systems and probably get some temporary fiscal relief. But until we focus reform efforts on where most of the money goes, which is healthcare delivery, we will remain stuck in a revolving door of near disaster and narrow escapes. To get to the point where all people have access to high-quality healthcare, affordably, we must focus our attention on how the healthcare delivery system determines costs and quality. Then we need to change that delivery model entirely.

In fact, hospitals, physicians, and nurses—all of healthcare—must change. First, we must emphasize the science of medicine over the art. This means turning to evidence-based medicine, which is already underway in some sectors. But we are also talking about evidence-based delivery, work that has barely begun.

In the hospitals and clinics of the ThedaCare medical system in Wisconsin's Fox River Valley, we have learned that every medical act is a series of steps that can be examined and improved. By investigating these steps, and the path that patients take through our hospitals and clinics, we have learned to identify value from the patient's point of view and to start getting rid of the waste that clogs the system of healthcare delivery.

In doing this work, we have made life better for our patients. In 2002, for instance, mortality rate for coronary bypass surgery at ThedaCare was nearly 4%—about 12 deaths per year.[2] After several improvement projects in cardiac surgery over seven years, in which we typically removed 40% of wasted time and effort with each pass, cardiac mortality was reduced to near zero.[3] Also, a patient's average time spent in hospital fell from 6.3 days to 4.9 and the cost of a coronary bypass declined 22%. Teamwork like this has saved us more than $27 million and ThedaCare has passed those savings along, becoming the overall lowest-price healthcare provider in Wisconsin.[4]

Seven years in to the revolution at ThedaCare, a not-for-profit system of hospitals, clinics, nursing homes, and other services that offers cradle-to-grave care, we have also doubled our operating margin. We have become better custodians of the public health dollar.

What we have discovered over the course of this work is that a different kind of healthcare is possible—care that is patient-focused, with less waste and cost and better medical outcomes. Using the improvement model popularized by the Toyota Production System,[5] we have arrived at *lean healthcare* and three organizing principles—focus on patients, value, and time—that are built upon a foundation of continuous improvement and respect for people. We have learned how to apply these principles to a large medical system with striking results.

2. Nationally, mortality rates for cardiac bypass surgery ranged between 3.44% and 2.3% from 1993 to 2003, with the numbers generally improving, according to the U.S. Department of Health and Human Service's Agency for Healthcare Research and Quality.

3. Out of ThedaCare's 350 cardiac patients in 2009, there was one death attributable to coronary bypass surgery.

4. Wisconsin Hospital Association. View full results at www.wipricepoint.org

5. The Toyota Production System has been studied and replicated all over the world by companies in every industry striving to produce better-quality products with fewer resources. In 2010, Toyota suffered multiple setbacks for failing to quickly address quality problems, a core tenet of the Toyota Production System. We do not consider this a repudiation of Toyota's principles, but instead a reminder of the consequences of failing to adhere to those principles.

By starting with the value being delivered to patients and thinking carefully about the delivery process for creating this value, we have proved that it is possible to enhance patient experiences while dramatically improving medical outcomes and lowering costs. Finally, we have distilled our experiments into an action plan that the senior management team of any healthcare organization can follow to achieve similar results.

One of us, John Toussaint, practiced internal medicine for 17 years before serving as chief medical officer and then chief executive officer of ThedaCare. He is now president of the ThedaCare Center for Healthcare Value. Co-author Roger Gerard, ThedaCare's chief learning officer, has been deeply involved in organizational development and change-management issues within this large organization for 19 years. We are stepping forward, encouraging others to expand on the work we have done, because we believe this is the path we must take to get better care to more people.

In telling our story, we sometimes have adopted an unusual voice. We have worked together in the same organization for many years but sometimes on different issues from different points of view. So in the pages ahead when we say *we*, we mean John and Roger. And when we say *John* or *Roger*, we are indicating that one of us took the lead in some activity.

Throughout this book, we are speaking directly to the people involved with delivering healthcare. We do not mean to suggest, however, that the external environment of healthcare—payment systems, insurance coverage, and regulations—does not need to be overhauled. It is a badly broken system requiring major surgery. But we are convinced that the healthcare debate needs to start from a deep understanding of how healthcare value is actually delivered.

This is an understanding we all need—policy makers and patients, as well as medical professionals. We all have a role to play in reforming healthcare. Caregivers need to rethink their priorities and remake their working environments. Lawmakers need to rewrite the rules to ensure that value is rewarded instead of waste. And patients must understand how healthcare works in order to demand truly effective change.

Only when we all have clear insight into the work going on inside the black box can useful reforms be crafted. We will return to this point in the concluding pages with a few additional thoughts about the health-care policy debates ahead. But for now let's begin where we started 10 years ago: with the patient, at the point of care.

Part **I**

Lean Healthcare
Process

Chapter 1

Discovering the Principles of Lean Healthcare

T hedaCare is a pretty typical, mid-sized, cradle-to-grave, not-for-profit healthcare provider. It consists of two major hospitals, Appleton and Theda Clark medical centers, plus rural hospitals, 20 primary-care offices, a network of specialists, nursing homes, assisted-living facilities and hospice care, inpatient and outpatient psychiatric care, physical therapy, and home health services. In all, ThedaCare facilities get more than 20,000 hospital admissions every year and the organization is the largest employer in northeast Wisconsin with about 5,500 people on staff.

Wisconsin's Fox Valley, which runs north of Lake Winnebago and is home to about half a million people, has a fairly homogenous population. There are a lot of dairy farmers and paper-mill workers and the area still has a good bit of light industry. Doctors see diabetes and hypertension, but few gunshot wounds.

Back in 2002, when ThedaCare began this transformation to lean healthcare, it was considered a very good organization. The National Committee for Quality Assurance, which accredits health plans in the United States, reports annually on which plans have the best Health

Employer Data Information Sets (HEDIS). Essentially, this is a measure of how well a health plan's doctors do on a series of quality-of-care measures. For instance, HEDIS scores look at whether patients are getting regular screenings for cervical or prostate cancers, if cholesterol levels and blood pressures are improving among heart patients. In 2000 and 2001, ThedaCare's health maintenance organization had the best HEDIS scores in the nation.[6]

Compared to other healthcare organizations ThedaCare was very good; the nation's best on one important measure. But is this how hospitals and physicians should measure quality when lives are at stake—*comparatively*?

The truth was, ThedaCare's medical professionals were causing unnecessary harm to patients, both through acts of omission and commission. Physicians, nurses, and administrators were focused on what worked for them instead of what worked for the patient. People recognized that timeliness of treatment was a major concern, but nobody was trying to improve care-delivery time in any organized way.

With every improvement, it seemed, ThedaCare also regressed. To understand why and how, let's go back to 1987, when John was chief of medicine, as a series of blood sugar spikes was occurring in the Intensive Care Unit at Appleton Medical Center.

These spikes were happening to the sickest patients in ICU, people with failed digestive systems who needed to be fed through an intravenous catheter. To keep their bodies alive and fighting, these patients receive a highly concentrated solution of glucose and vitamins through a catheter inserted into a major vein in the chest or neck. This solution, called parenteral nutrition, is caustic and delicately balanced.

---

6. That health maintenance organization, Touchpoint, has since been sold. ThedaCare now publicly reports its quality metrics through the Wisconsin Collaborative for Healthcare Quality, wchq.org.

That year, several parenteral nutrition patients suffered life-threatening spikes in their glucose levels. One person died. Each case was presented to the doctors' peer-review committee and finally John, in his role as chief of medicine, did a broader case review of all patients receiving parenteral nutrition. At the time, 30 or 40 patients required parenteral nutrition every month and there was little consistency as to solutions —or recipes—ordered by individual doctors. Every month, five or six patients had trauma related to their recipes. Diabetics were given inappropriate glucose concentrations; there were cases of dehydration and infection.

Yet the hospital's on-staff nutritionist, who spent years developing an expertise with these solutions, was treated like a waitress taking orders. She saw doctors prescribing solutions that she knew were ill advised, but could do little except write politely worded disagreements in the patients' charts. She suggested, she recommended, but could only fulfill doctors' orders.

After an exhaustive chart review, John sat down with the nutritionist to understand the issues. Together, they wrote a common protocol for parenteral nutrition—a kind of template for doctors to use when ordering the solution—and then presented it to the committee of peers. In that peer-review meeting, the protocol was denounced as "cookbook medicine" by doctors who said it would undermine their autonomy. It was dismissed.

As chief of the Medicine Department, John had one advantage over his colleagues: he set the monthly peer-review agenda. And for three months, the problem with parenteral nutrition was the only item on that agenda. He led doctors through the case histories, talked through the logic of the protocols. Finally, when it was clear John was not giving up, the doctors voted 12-11 to use the protocol.

Six months later, incidents of high blood sugar among ICU patients receiving the nutrition dropped from about five per month to zero. From five life-threatening emergencies in the ICUs of two urban hospitals each month to none.

It was a step toward evidence-based medicine and a powerful lesson in the use of standards to save lives and deliver better healthcare. But it was not tied to any sustainable method for improvement. Over time, some doctors forgot about the protocol. Newer doctors did not utilize the nutritionist, who was never given real authority or mandate. Although incidents of blood sugar spikes became rare, the perfect record proved impossible to sustain.

In 2000, after eight years of similar efforts to improve clinical performance without a systematic method, John left his role as chief medical officer to accept responsibility as ThedaCare's chief executive officer. Now determined to make radical change, as opposed to incremental or temporary improvement, he knew that he needed a structured improvement program. But he had never seen one tried in medicine that he could fully support. So with a small team of colleagues, he went looking outside healthcare for improvement strategies and, in 2002, they found themselves learning to make snow blowers.

The Factory as Teacher

A snow blower is not a particularly sensitive piece of equipment. It sucks snow in, mixes it with air, and blows the mix out in a concentrated rush. Making one does not involve the variables of diabetes treatment or childbirth. And most of the senior executives who went with John to that snow blower factory thought they knew something of the theories and practices of manufacturing. But at the Ariens, Inc. snow blower factory in Brillion, WI, everything was different from what they expected.

First, there was no assembly line. Employees had arranged the necessary manufacturing machines into small, U-shaped cells for each family of products and were working cooperatively to make each snow blower in one continuous flow of work. The employees knew how many snow blowers were needed, if there were any quality issues, and how to diagnose problems. They did not mouth words about teamwork; they worked collaboratively. And they were making more snow blowers at lower cost than previously—rescuing Ariens from the brink of bankruptcy. At the snow blower factory, ThedaCare doctors, nurses, and managers learned hands-on about the continuous-improvement methods of the Toyota Production System.

Before Toyota started exporting its laughably small cars in the 1970s, Americans expected cars to require a lot of maintenance. Repair bills were factored into the cost of owning a car—even brand new. Toyota changed that, providing reliability even on less expensive models. Manufacturers and academics went to Japan to learn the secret and many came back to spread the word. The word they chose to describe Toyota concepts such as just-in-time production and customer-pull and quality at the source was *lean*.

Those early converts were in for a hard slog against the idea of American exceptionalism, however—after all, the United States had the biggest and best car companies in the world—and for three decades, the concepts of lean manufacturing did not spread much past the manufacturing sector, even as some manufacturers recorded double-digit productivity using lean methods.

Among the snow blowers, and in subsequent visits to other factories employing the Toyota Production System, ThedaCare's doctors and administrators learned the core concepts of lean manufacturing: Recognize waste in all its manifestations and eliminate it; create one-piece flow to speed the product from start to finish and improve continuously; make sure every action and intention is focused on the needs of the customer.

For many on ThedaCare's original exploratory team, it felt as though a new world was being unveiled. Sick people were not snow blowers. The snow blowers were in many ways treated better. Work on each snow blower was designed to happen efficiently, without waiting between procedures, and with every employee understanding his or her role. Quality had improved dramatically. There was a lot to learn on that shop floor.

As the team made additional trips and returned to ThedaCare to reflect on the principles of lean healthcare, a creative adaptation of the lean principles discovered in manufacturing began to emerge.

Core Principles

In the end, we simplified what we learned into the fundamental principles of lean healthcare: Focus on patients, value, and time, using continuous improvement and respect for people as the foundation. In other words:

Focus on patients (not the hospital or staff) and design care
around them.

Identify value for the patient and get rid of everything else (waste).

Minimize time to treatment and through its course.

Focusing on patients, value, and time is the game plan for everything we do; continuous improvement and respect for people is the vehicle for change. The term "continuous improvement" is used today in various ways, but ThedaCare uses it to mean seeking out ways to change and improve work practices every day in every area. In other words, let no dogma go unchallenged.

While continuous improvement is always necessary, it is never easy. Job descriptions change and authority is challenged. Long-cherished ideas about the right way to work get punched like a piñata. Yet, ThedaCare has zealously and continuously embraced the principles of lean healthcare and the foundation necessary to achieve it since 2002. How has this been possible in an organization with a long history of improvement, followed by regression?

True North

In the daily rush of running hospitals and making people well, these principles can be easily forgotten. Who has time to worry about concepts when there are robotic surgical techniques to learn and new clinics to pay for? The solution is clear, simple, visual measurements that everyone can see.

In ThedaCare's continuous-improvement environment, the focus on lean principles and improvement is maintained through measurement. The specific metrics change from one hospital or business office to the next, but the measurements are always focused on safety, quality, people, delivery, and cost.

In every unit and hospital, a large board displays the data that is most relevant to the improvement work for that unit, plus the metrics that are critical to ThedaCare as a whole. For instance, a unit in the ICU that has recently improved patient safety by removing all trailing electrical cords from the floor will be tracking incidents of patient falls closely. But supervisors will also be tracking data to illustrate how the unit is doing in terms of quality, staff engagement, delivery, and cost. As an organization, ThedaCare has identified core "true north" metrics around patient satisfaction and safety, including mortality and medical error, employee engagement, productivity, and financial stewardship. (More on that later.) Those metrics are always on display in a central conference room, and all senior managers are presented with the newest numbers and trends once a month. It may seem like a lot of charts and numbers to keep current, but it is critical work because, without an accurate picture of reality, it is impossible to improve and sustain improvements.

Eliminating practices that take time and do not add value often mean slaughtering—or at least gently shoving aside—some sacred cows. And most of these cows do not go gently. Only when armed with accurate, trusted data can improvement teams make a case for change.

Please Note

To nonmedical readers: As we present the principles and foundations of lean healthcare in these next chapters, you will encounter more than one bloody mess. Our intention is not to shock. But medicine is not always pretty, even when practiced by a good organization like ThedaCare. The mess you will see in these pages is not unlike the mess to be found in every hospital in the country.

To our colleagues: We hope you will find the tools, the principles, and the impetus in these pages to help you deliver better, more cost effective healthcare—for your patients and for your staff. The average person goes to work every day seeking to do a job well. We all want progress, a sense of improvement. Most of us only need the right tools.

Lean healthcare is difficult and gratifying work, and it is the only method we have found to make long-term improvements stick.

Chapter 2

Focus on the Patient

I t was just after dinner on a bitterly cold night in March 2007 that Myrtle Bellis took a turn for the worse. Her skin grew pale and clammy, her heartbeat skipped and fluttered; she could not catch a full breath. As Myrtle lost and regained consciousness, her daughter Cindy telephoned for an ambulance and gathered up their coats.

Cindy Krueger followed a few minutes after the ambulance through a storm of snow and ice to Appleton Medical Center, certain that her 91-year-old mother was suffering from pneumonia. All the signs were there and it would be Myrtle's eleventh round with the disease. Cindy thought her mom just needed antibiotics, but she was not willing to take a risk with her mother's fragile health. After all, she was no doctor.

When she arrived at the Emergency Room, Cindy found her mother on a gurney, parked in a hallway, lying in her own waste. Myrtle had been taken for a CT scan where she had a bowel problem, and then she was simply returned to the emergency department to wait. Cindy asked for help cleaning her mother from people in the ER who were "too busy." An orderly finally arrived to transfer Myrtle to a hospital room and he helped Cindy maneuver her mother into a bathroom for cleanup.

Later, Myrtle was tucked into bed without diagnosis or treatment to wait until morning. Cindy drove home for a couple hours of sleep.

The treatment Myrtle received is one of the ugly truths that nobody in healthcare likes to face, but we must. In order to create meaningful change, everyone will have to look closely what happens to patients, especially in the worst moments.

Morning Rounds

In a medical unit—meaning nonsurgical, nonemergency—such as the one where Myrtle was admitted, doctors usually come to patients' rooms early in the morning. They check the chart for lab results, ask the patient a few questions if possible, write new orders, and leave. These physicians are known as hospitalists and they see a lot of chronic illness and elderly patients.

ThedaCare used to run medical units in this same way: hospitalists did rounds alone or with residents and students, wrote orders, and then depended on nurses assigned to that unit to carry out those hastily written instructions. Hospitalists and nurses were not assigned to patients; they were assigned to units and to weekly schedules. Some doctors were good about updating the electronic medical record quickly; some were not.

As Cindy Krueger recalls, four different physicians saw her mother during morning rounds over four days. One doctor thought he saw inconclusive evidence of pneumonia. The others believed it was probably something else—a bad cold or "just old age." Cindy was at her mother's bedside by 6 a.m. every day and, after one bad scare, began staying with Myrtle all day.

"My mother has diet-controlled diabetes. She doesn't take drugs," Cindy said. "The first day, though, a nurse came in with a needle full of insulin. I sent her away. Another time a nurse came in with syringe and said, 'This has got to go in her belly.' She told me it was [a blood thinner] because mother was bedridden. But mother wasn't bedridden at all. I had her up and down all the time.

"Finally, my mom was scared to be alone because nurses would come in with pills and when she asked what the pills were for, the nurses would just say, 'Something the doctor ordered.' They didn't seem to know *why* they were doing anything."

After four days, Cindy withdrew her mother from Appleton Medical Center. The following day, she took Myrtle to her regular doctor, who prescribed a round of antibiotics. Myrtle was feeling better within a week.

S.O.P.

The standard operating procedure in U.S. hospitals is such that anecdotes like this keep happening. An orderly is told that it is his job to deliver a patient on a gurney to the CT scan. A nurse's job is to deliver medication ordered by the doctor. Whose job is it to care for the patient?

Meanwhile, doctors are expected to drop in to a patient's room and the possibly complicated medical scenarios therein—perhaps the result of years of chronic illness—give the issue less than 15 minutes, get it right and move on. And then there is little consultation between the specialties. Healthcare professionals operate in virtual silos and with great authority. Heart doctors usually know little about bones; they leave that work to the orthopedic surgeons. Your cardiologist is not conferring with your urologist, and neither doctor is speaking to your psychiatrist. Likewise, a hospital laboratory has ineffective and scant communication with the pharmacy or internists.

Here is the ugly outcome of this silo working style: lack of communication and lack of focus on the patient, as a whole, results in misguided or contradicting orders and millions of incidents of medical harm every year.

"That's the way it used to be here and nobody liked it," said Jamie Dunham, RN, manager of the Collaborative Care unit at ThedaCare's Appleton Medical Center. "The doctors would come in and say something to the patient and then the nurse came along later, tried to read the doctor's notes and asked the patient, 'What did he say?' We were so task oriented—delivering medications and baths and drawing blood—we weren't really caring for the patient."

A New Way, Again

Realizing that ThedaCare needed change, leaders tried one improvement program after another over the course of many years. Most of the programs offered incrementally better results for a while, until everyone slid back into old habits.

In the 1990s, people seized on the idea of electronic medical records as the answer to doctors' information needs. With all records available at the touch of a button, the argument went, contradictions and miscommunication would evaporate.

In 1996, ThedaCare became one of the first healthcare systems in the world to make medical records available electronically and it was no panacea. All the waste in the system—such as redundancies and mistakes—was replicated electronically. Few doctors took the time to slog through screen after screen of seemingly irrelevant information. Physicians and nurses complained that time spent looking through records cut into face-time with patients.

Finally, it became clear that more than computerized records, patients needed individual and undivided attention. ThedaCare's leaders started thinking about breaking down the divisions between caregivers' specialties, divisions of labor, and habits of working to create a unified focus on the patient. Because this would require change of everyone involved, it was clear that hospital units needed a revolution instead of isolated, incremental adjustments.

Starting from Scratch

In early 2007, a core team of nurses, pharmacists, administrators, social workers, and physicians was assigned to work for six months on redesigning the inpatient care process—addressing the facility design, the work duties, and the specialized skills of everyone involved.[7] The team included Jamie Dunham, who had been agitating for change in nurses' working conditions, and others like her. Former patients and leaders from other industries—such as our friends from Ariens, the snow blower company—were invited to consult as well.

The makeover team was determined to burn down the old hospital model—one of medicine's most sacred cows—in order to engage all staff directly with patients. They used lean principles as a guide, but also redefined the model to become more patient-focused. This was in striking contrast to the traditional model of care in hospitals, where physicians control patient care, giving orders that are followed by all other caregivers who are not expected to provide input.

The team began by documenting the typical journey of a patient admitted to a hospital unit. By drawing a value-stream map that recorded every step taken by caregivers attending the patient, it soon became apparent that the activity surrounding the patient was a hectic, wasteful

---

7. This work was made possible in part by a Robert Wood Johnson Foundation grant administered by the Institute for Healthcare Improvement.

mess. Nurses were constantly hunting down and fetching supplies instead of using their skills and training at the patient's bedside. They were often out of the loop regarding patient needs. Doctors were not getting complete and accurate information, and were not consistent in communicating a plan of care. Pharmacists were so far removed from the action that they were rarely consulted at all. As a result, there were many medication errors. Each specialty was locked in its own silo.

To deal with the chaos, just about everyone was in the habit of making heroic saves. When a patient was harmed, managers would track the error to an individual and place blame, as if that was a solution. This was not unusual in American medicine; "shame and blame" is the most common form of addressing medical error in this country. Still, documenting the baseline performance to see what was actually happening to the patient on a unit floor, instead of what was supposed to be happening to the patient, was humbling for ThedaCare.

Over six months, the team collected data, dreamed up new ways to accomplish tasks, took turns playing different roles and kept asking, "How does this step benefit the patient?" They used cardboard and surplus equipment to mock up an idealized hospital room, and then a better hospital unit. At each step the team asked, "Does this task, done this way, serve the patient's needs?"

The Birth of Collaborative Care

The new unit, operational since late 2007, is essentially a large square, with all patient rooms facing an open meeting area where healthcare teams meet to confer on patient care. The new layout means that no patient is hidden away in a room down the hall, far from the nurses' station. Every patient room is visible from the central meeting area and each room has a large supply cabinet that is filled from outside the room—using a set of slide-out shelves accessed by a closet door just outside the patient's room—so as not to disturb the patient with housekeeping.

Each of those slide-out supply cabinets includes a secure drug box, stocked with the patient's medications. (Although some narcotics are kept in another secured location with tightly controlled access.) Pharmacy technicians, who resupply the drug boxes, use bar-code readers to double-check identity as they make their rounds. They also carry extra supplies on their carts to restock the shelves, so as not to waste a trip. The carts have become compact, rolling pharmacies. Because all supplies are situated near the patient's bed, nurses have stopped hunting and gathering throughout their shifts.

More important than architectural changes, Collaborative Care has completely altered the working lives of doctors, nurses, and pharmacists, making them full partners in patient care. Roles were redefined and new standards set.

Now, in the Collaborative Care unit, a nurse, physician, and pharmacist gather with the patient and family within 90 minutes of admission to develop a care plan. Everyone is involved in the discussion. The medical team is also together for morning rounds to check the care plan and modify it as needed. Nurses are never left with illegible orders. Instead, the nurse is part of the original discussions and knows how and why everything is happening.

"When you first graduate, you really want to be the perfect nurse— get to know your patients, explain things to them and make them comfortable. Then you get overwhelmed with tasks and everything starts slipping away," said Jamie Guth, a nurse in the Collaborative Care unit. "The first day I spent shadowing another nurse in Collaborative Care, I saw again the nurse I wanted to be."

Pharmacists, once hidden away in the basement pharmacy counting pills, have also become front-line caregivers. Besides joining in the initial consultation, the pharmacist attends morning rounds whenever possible. His or her presence at the patient's bedside addresses one of the most problematic issues in hospitals: medication reconciliation. This means reconciling the list of drugs the patient is actually taking with the list of drugs the patient should be taking—often prescribed by various doctors without consulting one another—with the drugs that doctors now think are needed. One of the most common errors made by staff is inadvertently omitting a drug the patient was taking at home during his or her hospital stay, according to the Institute for Healthcare Improvement. It is widely believed that medication reconciliation error is the root cause of most cases of patient harm. Yet the pharmacist is usually hidden away in a basement, counting pills without knowledge of their use.

On the floor of a Collaborative Care unit, the pharmacist enters a patient room pushing a computer cart, connected wirelessly to the hospital system, with two flat-screen monitors—looking like a two-headed monster. One screen shows the patient's current medications; the other has current lab results or new orders. Meeting with the patient in person, verifying current drug usage, and consulting with the doctor about new prescriptions has helped the team reduce medication reconciliation errors to zero for the past two and a half years.[8]

"We're seeing the patient now, not just the lab results or the doctor's orders. We're seeing the person and the response to drug therapies," said Charlotte Gutowski, Appleton Medical Center's lead pharmacist.

As one of the original Collaborative Care team members, Gutowski was particularly struck by patient complaints about being asked repeatedly for the list of their current medications—by clerks, nurses

8. Prior to Collaborative Care, hospital units at ThedaCare averaged 1.25 medication reconciliation errors per chart.

and doctors who were not, apparently, speaking to each other. Now, pharmacists are responsible for collecting that information and Gutowski finds herself spending quality time with patients—a lot of time, with some—making sure she knows every drug being taken at what dose and frequency. She calls it putting on her sleuth hat.

This means that pharmacists are no longer mere order-takers. They closely monitor kidney function to assess the patient's reactions to drugs and they consult with family members. They are full partners in care. Many doctors working in the Collaborative Care units, in fact, note in their prescriptions that the pharmacist is to decide dosage.

The pharmacist's cart, with its two-headed computer, is admittedly unwieldy and not a particularly elegant solution. But it is a good illustration of a lean healthcare ethos: make it better now; make it perfect later. Patients prefer that their medications are correct immediately. Elegance is secondary.

Foresight

The plan of care decided at the initial patient consultation goes beyond the usual "doctor's orders" in that it is not just prescriptive, it is predictive. In the old model, a doctor might order a drug and a laboratory test and move on. Now, the plan of care includes not just the drug, but also how long the patient is expected to stay on the drug, what lab tests should be ordered to check the drug's effects, and how the dosage might be changed based on lab results. The plan of care might include when and how much physical activity a patient should get, and how dietary habits might need to change over the predicted course of the hospital stay. And the plan always includes the patient's expected discharge date— also written on a board in the patient's room—so that all paperwork and appointments can be completed before that time.

So, the plan of care is an informed prediction of the course of a patient's hospital stay. There are many intersections along a patient's journey and a patient may encounter detours along the way. But foresight enables staff to plan ahead and cut down on the wasteful waiting that a patient often endures just before being discharged.

Having a unified plan of care also means that the physician is not the only one who knows what needs to happen. In Collaborative Care, a nurse takes over as case manager as soon as the plan is written and each nurse is assigned two or three patients to manage. As the patient moves through a series of "tollgates," spelled out in the plan of care, the nurse is responsible for ensuring that every clinical necessity happens before the next tollgate. For instance, the nurse will be sure that the dosage of a blood pressure medication known to cause dizziness is reduced before attempting to walk a patient down the hall. Nurses also use Milliman Guidelines, which are recognized conventions for the care of a wide range of medical conditions and chronic illnesses, to predict a patient's progress through care.[9]

Using the Milliman Guidelines plus the individualized plan of care, nurses are expected to stay alert to patient needs before they happen and to notify other team members if something—like new testing—needs to occur. The nurse maintains the master checklist, making sure key clinical criteria are met before the patient receives the next aspect of care. Airline pilots use a similar process to check that all systems are ready before their wheels leave the ground and before they land.

Like pharmacists, nurses in the Collaborative Care unit are full partners in patient care. Because they participate in all consultations, the nurse is cognizant of each step in a care sequence and can more confidently inform and educate patients and their families. Nurses also collect

---

9. Milliman Guidelines include benchmarks for beginning and ending standard, recognized therapies for medical conditions. Pneumonia or congestive heart failure, for instance, have guidelines that include giving certain drugs at specified times, and include expected length of stay in hospital.

and share information on the psychological and social needs and background of the patient. If the patient is grieving the loss of a spouse, for instance, or can only afford half of the prescribed drugs, everyone on the team can be informed.

These were new roles for nurses and physicians and sometimes there was friction before acceptance. Doctors are trained to be autocratic and firm in their decisions. Many nurses were attracted to their profession because they wanted to help, not lead. An Organizational Development team worked for weeks with staff in the mocked-up patient care unit, role playing and working through the repercussions of nurses directing doctors and orchestrating team approaches to care before real patients arrived in a real Collaborative Care unit.

Still, not everyone was comfortable with the new model, concedes Dr. Mark Hermans, administrative lead of the hospitalists[10] at Theda Clark and Appleton medical centers. As one of the original designers of the Collaborative Care model, Dr. Hermans knew that he was asking other physicians to accept a lot of change.

"Doctors are used to working independently, not having people right there in our thought processes. A team meeting is like being on stage," Dr. Hermans said. "Also, you're working with a group of colleagues that you're elevating, in terms of medical knowledge, and you have to be comfortable being challenged by your team as they learn more."

A few doctors did not appreciate the change and left ThedaCare for other opportunities. Most of the staff hospitalists stayed, however, and in extensive physician interviews after the pilot site had been operational for several months, doctors reported that the nurses in Collaborative Care were better informed, better at thinking on their feet, and more helpful to the doctors overall.

---

10. Hospitalists are general physicians, usually internists, who practice on the nonspecialized, nonsurgical medical units of a hospital.

New-patient admissions and morning rounds require more time in the new model, but improvement teams are shaving minutes off here and there. Rounds that took 30–40 minutes per patient early in the Collaborative Care unit's operation are now averaging 23–25 minutes. That is still more time than it takes for a single doctor to pop in, check on a patient and make his notes. Then again, doctors in Collaborative Care report fewer calls from nurses and pharmacists later in the day with questions about orders. That means fewer misunderstandings, headaches, and interruptions for the physician. It also means fewer errors, which touch off new rounds of work for everyone.

Lean thinkers in every industry put in this extra time at the beginning of a process and find that it pays big dividends down the line in terms of time savings and fewer errors. This is often referred to as building quality at the source.

The Change Routine

Instead of responding to hierarchy and heroically firefighting in an environment of shame and blame, Collaborative Care teams now meet in daily huddles to review any issues with patients or work flow. When problems arise such as a medication error or a patient fall, team members use PDSA (plan, do, study, act) cycles to determine what happened, find a corrective plan, implement it, and study the results on the process. Teams then create new standard work[11] or, if the change did not achieve the desired results, the PDSA cycle begins again. PDSAs are not drawn-out or academic exercises and are often completed in an afternoon. (*See Chapter 5 for a more complete description of PDSA.*)

---

11. Standard work is a step-by-step description of the actions and tools needed to complete a task. It is a foundation of continuous improvement, because a task cannot be changed and improved if we do not know how it was accomplished in the first place.

When errors occur now, instead of scrutinizing people, people study the process. Staff members write and rewrite standard work as they search for better methods and work sequences. As other lean organizations have discovered before ThedaCare, people are very rarely the problem. If there is an error, the fault is usually in the design and sequence of work.

The Results of Teamwork

Collaborative Care began with a pilot unit in late 2007. In the first two years of operation, 2,400 people were cared for in that unit, with dramatic improvement in patient satisfaction, quality performance, and reduced medication errors compared with similar hospital units. (*See Figure 1, Collaborative Care Results, in the Appendix.*)

Quality of pneumonia care, for instance, went from hitting 38% of the quality markers to achieving 95%, consistently. That means patients with pneumonia are now getting 95% of every possible need—as defined by a federal quality panel—cared for now instead of having those needs met less than two-fifths of the time.

Patients report being "very satisfied" with the total experience of their care while in hospital 90% of the time instead of 68%, and they are staying in hospital about three days instead of nearly four, on average. Overall, patients are receiving better medical outcomes in shorter stays.

Because the original Collaborative Care design team worked hard to remove wasted time, resources and energy from work sequences—and every improvement project cuts out more waste—cost of care in a Collaborative unit is now 30% less than a traditional unit. When ThedaCare board members were presented with this data, they decided to convert all hospital beds to Collaborative Care. This decision was projected to improve the buildings' net present value by 63%, or more than $25 million.[12] That means if there were two hospital towers built side-by-side, the Collaborative Care tower would be 63% more profitable than the traditional one. A new, eight-story hospital tower, opening in mid-summer 2010 at Appleton Medical Center, has been designed from the beginning as a Collaborative Care facility.

A second Collaborative Care unit has recently opened at Theda Clark Medical Center and there is an aggressive plan to convert all ThedaCare hospital beds to Collaborative Care by the end of 2011.

Better Care for Myrtle

A consultation with the doctor, nurse, and pharmacist assigned to her case within 90 minutes of Myrtle Bellis' admission to the medical unit would have done wonders for her care. If Myrtle's caregivers could have heard, all at once, from Myrtle's daughter that she had already suffered pneumonia 10 times and the current symptoms looked the same, it would have had a much larger impact.

If they had all decided together on the plan of care, Cindy could have rested easy, without worrying about what medications were being delivered to her mother. And if everyone from the orderlies to the surgeons knew that their primary job was to care for Myrtle and other patients like her—not transport her or give her tests or stop in and check her chart—then nobody would be left in a hallway with soiled pants.

This is the real benefit of Collaborative Care: communication between caregivers focused on the patient's well-being. Lower-cost healthcare is great, but medicine that puts the patient first is the goal.

---

12. Net present value is a mechanism for looking at financial performance of an investment over time. It takes into account the cost of money, based on a projected interest rate for that money, and then factors in cash flow and operating margin of the investment. If the net present value is positive it means the investment did better financially than if the money was simply kept in an investment vehicle at a fixed rate of return.

Finding Value

Providing excellent, waste-free healthcare is about more than teamwork and better communication, of course. It's about delivering only what is of value, quickly, by removing the many wasteful activities surrounding patients on their journey through diagnosis and treatment.

Medicine has become such a complicated maze of processes, paperwork, therapies, and specialties, however, that leaders and staff can easily lose sight of the definition of "value." Strip away layers of accumulated stuff—assumptions and policies and roles—and somewhere in there, you will find the real value being provided to the patient.

Most of the time, teams need to begin their search for true value with the most elementary of questions: What is "value" anyway?

Chapter **3**

Focus on Value

et's say you go to your doctor with a crushing headache. You will be asked to fill out a complete health history and answer a series of questions about your encounters with headaches. You will probably give blood and urine for tests relating to diabetes, possible infection, and thyroid malfunction. Next up is a CT scan in which X-rays and computers allow doctors to see cross-sections of your body and head. A sinus X-ray might be ordered, along with an eye exam or even a painful spinal tap.

The final answer: you have migraines. With a prescription in hand for a drug called a sumatriptan—which works for 70% of migraine sufferers—you are released.

Now ask yourself, what happened here that you are willing to pay for—the questions, the blood tests, the X-rays? Which part of your medical experience so far is of value?

When patients answer honestly, without undue reverence for the medical profession or regard for staff feelings, the answer is usually short and shocking. Nothing of value happened in that trip to the doctor because your head was still pounding as you left.

Strip away all the expectations about medicine and you will find that what people really want is not fancy tests, name-brand drugs, and flat-screen televisions in the waiting room. They want to be fixed—relieved from pain, returned to good health, assisted in delivering healthy babies. Everything else is noise and, very often, a waste of resources.

The Value Test

The goal of every lean practitioner is to find what is of value to the customer and deliver it reliably, while removing all extraneous acts and materials from the process. In the strictest definition, everything that is not of value is waste.

But how does one identify what is truly of value for the customer? Many healthcare professionals probably think having blood drawn is of value. In fact, most people do not enjoy being stuck with needles and would avoid it if they possibly could. They place a value on being accurately diagnosed, but not on the diagnostic tests, per se. Diagnostic tests fall under the category of "necessary nonvalue-creating," which can be a kind of holding pattern for waste—it is reluctantly accepted as necessary until some innovation comes along. On the day when blood can be "read" without pulling it out of the body, everyone will happily give up the needles. Until then, drawing blood is necessary but nonvalue-creating. Let's return to this later, however, and first define value.

In manufacturing, lean practitioners define value as something for which the customer is willing to pay. Looking at every aspect of production, they ask, would a customer pay for that? The customer would be willing to pay for the widget to be assembled and painted blue, for instance, but would not be willing to pay for a factory to overproduce widgets, truck them to a warehouse and store them until needed. Overproduction and storage are defined as waste.

In healthcare, looking for what is truly of value in a process is an emotionally loaded exercise. Not only do physicians embrace different methods and measures, there is often a good deal of ego invested in those methods. At ThedaCare, therefore, teams examining a process for improvement are continually reminded to consider the patient first.

Balloon Therapy

For instance, let's consider value from the point of view of a patient who is suffering a fairly common type of heart attack—an ST segment elevated myocardial infarction, or STEMI.[13] Many tests are administered and preliminary measures taken when a STEMI patient enters a hospital, but ThedaCare has identified value as the moment the patient's arteries are cleared of blockage and blood flow returns to normal.

In other words, the instant the block is cleared is the single moment of value. This value is on a sliding scale. The sooner blood flow returns to the patient's heart, the more heart muscle is saved from permanent damage and the more value is delivered. If too much time passes, the once-life-saving procedure is worthless. Time, doctors like to say, is muscle.

A peek inside the arteries of a typical STEMI patient may be instructive here. Let's say the patient is a 60-year-old man and time, cholesterol, fatty foods and heredity have conspired to create a buildup of plaque on the inside walls of his arteries. The opening has narrowed, but blood still flows. Then one day, a piece of this thickened arterial wall breaks off and platelets rush to the scene, just as they would to a skin abrasion, to form a clot and stop the bleeding. The clot stops blood flow completely, which kicks the nervous system into high alert and causes sweating and nausea. Pain shoots along his arm and jaw, and fluid

---

13. The ST segment is one part of the electrocardiogram (EKG) tracing that maps the overall electrical function of the heart. When this segment of the tracing is elevated from its baseline, it indicates a heart attack may be occurring.

stagnates in the lungs, causing shortness of breath. Starved of oxygen, heart cells begin dying and, after about five minutes, brain cells start dying off too. These cells are not replaceable. Enough heart cells die and tissue starts to die, causing the patient to develop scar tissue, which will be an impediment to future heart function. Exact timing for blockage-to-scar tissue differs from one patient to the next, but cardiologists agree that getting the block cleared within 90 minutes leaves the patient with a good chance of recovery.

Current clinical practice calls for this kind of blockage to be cleared by inserting a catheter into an artery in the groin and snaking it up to the heart where a balloon at the tip of the catheter is inflated, clearing away the plaque and platelets that were clogging the artery. This is the moment—when the balloon inflates, the clog is destroyed, and blood flow resumes—in which healthcare provides value to the patient.

Of course, certain procedures are necessary before the clog is cleared. Equipment must be purchased, maintained, and prepared; the right people need to be in place. The patient must be anesthetized, his groin area cleaned and clipped, the blockage pinpointed and other diagnostic exams performed. A patient history should be collected, including prior drug reactions, and most hospitals really do need insurance or payment information.

But which of these procedures are actually necessary? How much is waste? A conundrum of the value question is that some activities are necessary without being of value to the customer, as noted earlier. Billing is one example. Customers will not pay to be billed, but collecting the money is necessary in any business. Similarly, X-rays and blood tests do not achieve the end goal of pain relief, but may be necessary for diagnosis. Therefore, there are different levels of waste—from the obvious waste of sending someone in search of supplies that are not needed to performing an X-ray that reveals no actionable information.

Seeing the Flow

Learning to see waste in all of its manifestations is complicated because creating value for the patient always involves many steps often performed at many places. Fortunately, managers at Toyota many years ago devised an excellent tool for seeing value and waste in any human activity: the value-stream map.

A value-stream map identifies every task required to make a product or service as it moves through the organization. By documenting and carefully analyzing every step made during diagnosis and treatment, people involved in the work can pinpoint value and waste.

In early 2006, for instance, a team of about 10 people including doctors and nurses from Appleton Medical Center's cardiology and the emergency room, Emergency Medical Services (EMS) technicians, a fireman and administrators sat down in a room to document everything that happened to a Code STEMI patient from arrival in the ER to the moment a life-saving balloon was inflated in his vessel and blood flow returned. This is referred to as door-to-balloon time.

At that time, the American Heart Association, the American College of Cardiologists, and the Institute for Healthcare Improvement (IHI) all set 90 minutes or less as the door-to-balloon time goal. After 90 minutes, mortality markedly increases (i.e., more patients die), along with more incidence of damage to the heart muscle. Teams at Appleton and Theda Clark hospitals were hitting that 90-minute goal just 65% of the time.

"We were hurting people—damaging their heart muscles because we weren't responding fast enough," said Dan Collins, a registered nurse in the ER who helped lead the improvement team. "Look, we all have moms and dads and grandparents who live around here and come in through these doors. We want to make sure we are doing the best we can. We take it personal."

Using sticky notes on a conference room wall, the team documented every step from the moment a patient arrived in the ER with chest pains. A triage nurse evaluated the patient, took vital signs—blood pressure, pulse—and asked questions. That nurse then called another nurse to find an available room and alert the team to a possible heart emergency. The team in this case included a consulting cardiologist, a cardiac surgeon, catheter lab technicians, and nurses—although, not all of those team members would necessarily be notified right away.

The patient was then wheeled down the hall to another room and handed off to another nurse, helped out of his clothes and into a gown. This nurse might also start an IV line and draw blood for testing before attaching a series of electrodes to the patient's skin for electro-cardiography (EKG). This shows the heart's electrical activity and is the main diagnostic tool for heart problems.

Once the EKG was complete, the nurse collected the printout and might set it on a counter for the emergency room doctor to collect or, if the doctor were standing nearby, she might hand the EKG over for review. The emergency doctor might order more tests and wait 30 minutes for results and then, if she saw signs of a STEMI event, she would page the on-call cardiologist for consultation. If that cardiologist agreed with the diagnosis—following his own evaluation, of course— he would alert the clerk of a STEMI. The clerk used a staff roster and work schedules to make phone calls to the STEMI team, which brought in nurses, technicians, and doctors to perform the angioplasty. Once an available room was identified for surgery, the patient was moved and prepped for the procedure. (*See Figure 2, Intial STEMI Value-Stream Map, in the Appendix.*)

If this patient arrived in the middle of the night, he might wait 20 minutes for the on-call consulting cardiologist to get out of bed, come to the hospital and confirm the emergency doctor's diagnosis, and then wait another 20 minutes for the cath team—including the interventional cardiologist—to arrive, ready to operate. All the while his heart would be dying, cell by cell.

For every sticky note on the wall documenting a step in this lengthy process, the team considered the step's value and affixed a red dot for waste or a green dot, for value.

The Five Whys

Of course, determining "value" and "waste" for each step is not a simple task. Many ingrained habits take on the patina of value, simply because the actions are so often repeated. Looking at a habit and calling it "waste" usually means busting a few paradigms and for that, special tools are required. One of the simpler tools is to become unabashedly curious and, for every task or roadblock, ask "why." Then ask "why" four more times, drilling down through the initial "easy answers" until arriving at an actionable response.

Let's start with the problem of a STEMI patient's waiting time in the emergency room.

1. Why is the patient waiting? Because a cardiology consultation is needed.

2. Why the consult? Because the cardiologists say they must be the ones to diagnose a STEMI event.

3. Why are cardiologists needed? Because the cardiologists do not trust the emergency doctors to accurately diagnose a STEMI.

4. Why the distrust? Because emergency doctors have not been specifically trained to recognize a STEMI event.

5. Why? There is no standardized process to diagnose a STEMI event.

Looked at this way, the team wonders if the wait on a cardiology consultation can be eliminated by developing a standardized process by which those present in the emergency room can recognize and accurately diagnose a STEMI event, particularly if clear instructions were written and posted for all to see.

For this bit of log-jamming waste to be eliminated, however, cardiologists had to be convinced that others could make an accurate diagnosis. Fortunately, the Code STEMI team found a nearby hospital that had already eliminated the cardiology consultation.

In 2005, Gundersen Lutheran Medical Center in La Crosse, WI had the best door-to-balloon time in Wisconsin. One of the chief break-throughs in achieving this performance had been eliminating the cardiology "middle-man." The Code STEMI team went to Gundersen to see how the other team did it and, after a round of close questioning and plenty of discussion between cardiologists and emergency physicians, the improvement team had a clear picture of the problem.

Dr. Peter Ackell, an Appleton Medical Center cardiologist who was on the improvement team, explains it this way: people tend to get sick in the middle of the night. For years, emergency doctors had been calling cardiologists at 2 a.m. or 4 a.m. and were often subjected to grumpy, abrupt questions. Emergency doctors thought of cardiologists as short-tempered and imperious. Cardiologists thought of emergency doctors as those people that woke them up in the middle of the night, sometimes with false alarms. Could they be trusted to make the right diagnosis?

To get rid of the "middle-man" consultation, cardiologists needed to agree to let emergency physicians make the diagnosis that would roust the cath team—surgeon, nurses, and technicians—out of bed on a moment's notice. Emergency room doctors had to prove they could do this without false alarms or missed diagnoses.

"It was hard for us to relinquish control, absolutely. We worried about false alarms and talked through a lot of stuff," Dr. Ackell said. "As a result, though, the relationship between cardiologists and ER doctors has really improved."

Waste Removal

In early 2006, following the trip to Gundersen, the team conducted a one-week Rapid Improvement Event (RIE) at Appleton Medical Center, questioning every step in the process between door and balloon and eliminating the cardiology consultation. (RIEs are based on Toyota's concept of continuous improvement, called *kaizen*,[14] and are an important part of creating change at ThedaCare. There will be more complete descriptions of these events in coming chapters.)

Over the next 12 months, the Code STEMI team had weekly meetings and pored over the door-to-balloon time for every STEMI patient, looking for answers as to why some patients progressed quickly and others stumbled. If the team saw room for improvement—which was often—members devised new paths, wrote new standard work, and studied the sequence again.

Instead of relying on clerks to juggle the roster and staff contact sheets to figure out who to call, the first phone call now made after a patient walks in the door complaining of chest pains is to a dedicated line in the emergency room. Anyone who picks up that call can trigger automated calls to the ER physician, cardiologist, catheter lab technicians, and nurses warning of a possible STEMI.

And because the pivotal diagnostic test for a STEMI patient is the EKG, every bit of business between the door and the test has been removed. Today, if a patient walks in complaining of chest pains, he is

---

14. Kaizen is from the Japanese symbols meaning "change" and "good." It is usually translated as "change for the better."

immediately wheeled back to a dedicated room and met by a nurse with an EKG machine. Questions are usually asked and answered while the patient is en route and the EKG is hooked up immediately. A nurse then takes the printout, places it in the ER doctor's hand, and awaits instruction.

Meanwhile, another nurse is getting vital signs, starting IV lines, giving aspirin, and performing other important support tasks. Every medication that a STEMI patient needs—including aspirin, a beta-blocker, and a blood thinner—is stored in a kit box that a nurse grabs on her way into the room.

If the ER doctor sees a STEMI event on the EKG printout, the cath team—operating cardiologist, nurses, technician—is immediately paged and has 20 minutes to arrive, ready to perform an angioplasty. (*See Figure 3, Improved STEMI Value-Stream Map, in the Appendix.*)

After the first Rapid Improvement Event at Appleton Medical Center, the change was profound: no local STEMI case missed the 90-minute mark on door-to-balloon time. Cardiologists at Theda Clark in Neenah agitated to begin using the new work methods immediately. The two hospitals now have an average door-to-balloon time of 37 minutes, and an ongoing competition between the hospitals is helping keep everyone focused on getting the patient's vessels cleared more quickly.

ThedaCare covers a large swath of northeast Wisconsin and treats about three dozen STEMI patients every year. In the three years since that first week-long improvement event, there have been just three cases in which a STEMI patient landed in a cardiac catheterization lab more than 90 minutes after ThedaCare's initial contact. Those "outlier" cases led employees to study the problems of transporting emergency cases across great distances, even as cardiologists were pushing to bring the new work sequences to the six rural hospitals that ThedaCare works with.

Using lean principles, the teams devised new systems that now consistently deliver patients for angioplasty in less than 90 minutes—including time in ambulances and helicopters.

Because the Code STEMI process, including immediate EKG, is followed for every person who complains of chest pains, Dr. Ackell also believes that emergency room staff has captured more people —especially women and people with atypical symptoms—who are having a heart attack. And the cardiologists' fear that they would be dragged out of bed in the middle of the night for repeated false alarms by emergency room doctors? There have been two false alarms in three years. The doctors seem satisfied with the price paid for saving more hearts.

The Value-Stream Lesson

ThedaCare employees now map the value stream of every process that is being studied, looking for the moment of value for the patient, and the waste surrounding that value. Looking closely at work sequences, people now ask bigger questions. Should pharmacists be in the pharmacy? Or should they be at the bedside with the nursing staff, dealing with the pharmacological needs of the patient as part of a team? Should all testing be centralized in one lab? Would it better serve patients to perform simple, routine tests at bedside or in the patient care unit? Should housekeepers report to a centralized environmental services department or to the business unit manager where the work is being done, as part of the care team?

All of these questions and more are being addressed in team meetings every week, often with surprising results. There are no right answers or everlasting solutions, only incremental improvements to be tested and implemented as employees get closer to the goal of identifying what is of value to the patient, then delivering it reliably.

Diagnosed by the Driver

Because lean healthcare requires a restless pursuit of improvement, the most persistent question after the 5 Whys should be, "Why not?"

Why not trust emergency room doctors to diagnose a heart attack? If the patient is on a farm far from the hospital, why not trust the ambulance driver to administer and read an EKG?

If you visit a farm in the beautiful rolling hills of Valders, WI, for instance, and develop a clutching chest pain after the welcoming bratwurst fry, your ambulance driver can set up and administer an EKG, diagnose your ST segment elevated myocardial infarction, alert the team, and take you immediately to the helicopter and the flight to Appleton Medical Center for delivery straight to the cath lab.

If your driver is not trained to diagnose your STEMI, he will soon be able to transmit EKG results to the ER for diagnosis. And still, you will go from brat to balloon in under 90 minutes.

Applying the Lessons

Having learned to see the waste lurking in the work sequence around diagnosis and treatment of a STEMI event, where time is critical and hearts are at risk, one can begin to see the possibilities for applying these principles to the migraine that began this chapter.

Begin by asking, which diagnostic test is the most important? Does the answer change based on factors such as gender, age, and weight? Identify the critical test for diagnosing the largest fraction of such cases and push it to the front of the line. And since there is a known treatment—the sumatriptan family of drugs—that works on 70% of such cases with minimal side effects, why not administer the drug immediately in the doctor's office? The results are instantaneous.

Weigh this extra step in the care sequence against the safety risk of sending a patient with a blinding headache to the drugstore and then home, or scheduling expensive and unnecessary tests.

ThedaCare has also applied this work to stroke cases, because time isn't only muscle. As the next chapter shows, time is also brain when doctors are racing the clock to save cognitive function during a stroke.

Time is so critical in medicine that you may be surprised that it is not the first principle of lean healthcare. There is a difference, however, between hectic activity spent on tasks that are not creating value and patient-focused work that speeds care providers to the most valuable actions.

It is true that time is of the essence, but only in the right context.

Chapter 4

Minimize Time

Everything seemed to be running so smoothly that morning. A peach pie was already in the oven, the beefsteak was in marinade, and fresh beets were boiling on the stove. Standing at the kitchen sink, with her husband of 46 years beside her making a sandwich for lunch, Lee Parker was satisfied everything would be ready for the evening's dinner party.

And then she had the most curious feeling. It was as if her left arm was fading or being erased, pixel by pixel. She looked for her arm, certain that it would be going or gone, and saw it hanging at her side. Just hanging there. Her left leg weakened suddenly and buckled, pulling her body heavily into the counter. John Parker put down his sandwich, asked Lee if she was all right. Her words came out sloppy: "No, I don't think so."

It was 12:45 p.m. and a small blood vessel in a right branch off her middle cerebral artery had just slammed shut, probably blocked by a bit of plaque. Blood flow to the region upstream was cut off and, without oxygen pumping through the arteries, brain cells were beginning to die off at a rate of about 1.9 million per minute.[15]

---

15. http://ehealthvirginia.org/newsstroke/LossRateOfNeuronsToStroke.pdf

The next hour would be the most critical 60 minutes of Lee's life. Someone dies of stroke every 45 seconds in the United States. It is the third leading cause of death and the number-one cause of serious, long-term disability.[16] John grabbed a chair, set Lee on it, and called 911. The Appleton Fire Department and emergency medical technicians, responding from the Number 6 Station just blocks away, were there within five minutes. Struggling to form words and push them out of her mouth, Lee asked the emergency technicians to turn off the stove.

Lee still remembers looking out of the ambulance window as it sped to Theda Clark Medical Center, 10 miles away in Neenah, WI. They were going so fast, the trees were all a blur.

Lee was suffering an ischemic stroke, which is much like a heart attack in that a blood vessel becomes blocked and starves surrounding tissue of oxygen. Treatments include drug therapy or using a catheter inserted into the groin and fed up through an artery into the brain to suck out or grab and pull out the clot. Time to treatment is the most critical factor in a patient's chance for recovery and that makes the Stroke Center at Theda Clark the perfect place to illustrate lean healthcare's third principle: Minimize Time.

Gold Medal Care

In the United States, the mortality rate for all types of stroke is about 18% annually.[17] At ThedaCare in 2007, stroke mortality hit a low 8.8% and Theda Clark hospital, where most stroke patients are seen, was awarded Gold Medal status by the American Stroke Association. But here is what neurologists and nurses in the Stroke Center saw in 2009

---

16. http://www.strokecenter.org/patients/stats.htm
17. The American Heart Association, "Heart Disease and Stroke Statistics Update," final through 2005.

when they carefully examined the stroke diagnosis and treatment process: time-to-treatment in the stroke center was inconsistent and too many patients were dying.

Kristin Randall, coordinator of Theda Clark's Stroke Center, and her colleagues heard about the work being done to improve the outcome of heart attack cases and saw the parallels. So, in 2009 she joined forces with the lean experts from the ThedaCare Improvement System and put together a team to study the process.

Just as in heart attack care, the first and most important task in caring for a stroke victim is getting a picture of exactly what is happening inside the body. For strokes, the picture needed is a CT scan. National organizations like the Stroke Association and the Brain Attack Coalition set guidelines stating that a CT scan should be completed within 25 minutes of a patient entering the hospital doors and the scan should be read within 45 minutes.

Randall and her team found that at Theda Clark, 51% of patients were being scanned within 25 minutes and just 36% had a scan read within 45. And this was a Gold Medal facility.

The team assembled a value-stream map that soon showed why. After a patient arrived, people waited while a respiratory therapist was called to insert the 18-gauge IV needle required to inject a contrasting fluid into the bloodstream before a CT scan. Patients often waited next for an EKG to be done, for the stroke-specific CT scanner to be cleared of nonemergency cases, and while several phone calls were made to alert many departments. Lab work, which takes two minutes to process, was not always labeled as a priority and ended up in a laboratory queue.

"We were waiting for everything, for each task," Randall said.

Lee Parker remembers arriving at the Stroke Center in September 2008 and being surrounded by busy hands while a doctor spoke gently in her ear, telling her everything that was happening. She had no concept of waiting, only a far off sense of dread.

When Everything Worked

One spring morning in 2009, a 40-year-old woman was working in her office when the right side of her face suddenly fell. Paralysis of her entire right side quickly followed. She arrived at Theda Clark via ambulance at 9:49 a.m., 45 minutes after her symptoms began, and just at the right time for the Stroke Center's improvement team to observe and map the action. What followed was a both a command performance and an illustration of a classic process failure.

A respiratory therapist was there immediately with the 18-gauge needle required to inject the contrast fluid; blood was drawn for the kidney function test necessary before a CT scan. Under the watchful eyes of the improvement team, vital statistics were taken, an EKG was given, an IV was started and the patient was in the CT scanner at 9:55 a.m., six minutes after she arrived. Results were available at 10:20 and doctors determined the woman was eligible for the clot-busting drug therapy, tissue plasminogen activator (tPA).

So far, so good. The neurologist wrote an order for tPA and faxed it to the pharmacy, where the powerful, carefully calibrated medication takes 20 minutes to mix. When complete, the drug was expedited to the patient's room where the improvement team was still observing. They watched as the drug was delivered to a shelf in the patient's room and then left to wait while X-ray technicians claimed the patient in order to get chest X-rays.

Time is brain.

There are about 100 billion nerve cells, or neurons, in the average human forebrain.[18] Every minute that the patient's vessel was blocked meant the death of 1.9 million neurons and 14 billion synapses.[19] The X-ray, Randall said later, should have waited while tPA was administered to break the clot.

Despite unnecessary waiting, both this patient and Lee Parker got the necessary drugs within an hour of arriving at the hospital and began moving and feeling their limbs again within two hours. Lee's paralysis was gone in 20 minutes. These were two good outcomes in a Gold Medal unit. The question that troubled Randall after careful observation of the process was whether every patient, arriving at any time of day or night, could expect the same.

Defining Waste

As the team dug further into the stroke emergency work sequence, they discovered that the medical outcomes for Lee Parker and the 40-year-old patient were good—the result of dedicated, trained medical personnel working together—but overall, the hospital's response to stroke care was not reliable or repeatable. To get to reliable and repeatable, the improvement team would have to look hard at what every team member was doing at every moment and decide what was waste and what was of value. In particular, they wanted to find any business that wasted time.

This is a tricky bit of work. Those who look at the individual steps of a person's jobs—which are collectively the content of his or her working life—and pass value judgments risk demoralizing the staff member. Toyota engineers understood this when they set out to

---

18. The number of neurons in the human brain has been estimated at 10 billion and 100 billion, with the larger number now more widely accepted. Each of those neurons has about 7,000 synaptic connections to other neurons.
19. Synapses are the electrical connections between neurons and it is estimated that humans have more than 100 trillion synapses in the brain. Still, we don't want to be losing too many.

create the definitive list of wastes. They wanted to help employees recognize that tasks were either creating value or waste, instead of being told that their task was now deemed "worthless." Lean facilitators emphasize that it is the task being judged, not the person.

It was not difficult to adapt the Toyota Production System's "Seven Wastes" to healthcare. In fact, much of this material seems intuitive. ThedaCare also includes an eighth waste: talent.

The Eight Wastes of Lean Healthcare

1. *Defect*: making errors, correcting errors, inspecting work already done for error

2. *Waiting*: for test results to be delivered, for an appointment, for a bed, for release paperwork

3. *Motion*: searching for supplies, fetching drugs from another room, looking for proper forms

4. *Transportation*: taking patients through miles of corridors, from one test to the next unnecessarily, transferring patients to new rooms or units, carrying trays of tools between rooms

5. *Overproduction*: excessive diagnostic testing, unnecessary treatment

6. *Overprocessing*: a patient being asked the same question three times, unnecessary forms; nurses writing everything in a chart instead of noting exceptions

7. *Inventory* (too much or too little): overstocked drugs expiring on the shelf, under-stocked surgical supplies delaying procedures while staff goes in search of needed items

8. *Talent*: failing to listen to employee ideas for improvement, failure to train emergency technicians and doctors in new diagnostic techniques

While waiting is only one of the eight wastes of lean healthcare, it has such an outsized impact on patient outcomes, patient and staff engagement, and cost that ThedaCare recognized the need to make this waste a principle of its own: Minimize Time.

So, waiting is a waste, and minimizing time is one of the main goals —along with focusing on the patient and identifying value—of every improvement project. Teaching every ThedaCare employee to recognize the eight wastes and help eradicate them is also a goal of team projects.

Waste Steals Time

Waste is expensive. Just imagine if every hospital and physician practice could recoup the amount of money wasted on discarding out-of-date drugs, settling lawsuits for error, or performing unnecessary diagnostic tests. Fortunes would be reversed overnight. Maybe the word "healthcare" would not always be followed by "crisis."

Money is not the most important element that waste steals, however. The most important, from the patient's perspective, is time and health. Time is muscle; time is brain. Faster treatment means quicker, more complete recovery.

After the Stroke Center's improvement team completed the initial time studies and mapped the care sequence for stroke victims, the team held a one-week Rapid Improvement Event to decide how the process should be changed, and then change it. These week-long events, in which a small team of doctors, nurses, clerks, patients, and outsiders make physical changes to layouts and to job descriptions, is at the heart of lean healthcare's energy and excitement. We will describe these events more thoroughly in the next chapter; for now, let's focus on how the team's work bought time for stroke patients.

Spaghetti

Stroke patients are like snowflakes; no two are identical. When the team first began documenting the stroke care sequence, it also looked like snowflakes, with no two Code Stroke sequences being the same.

Depending on an emergency technician's training and inclination, an IV line would or would not be started before arrival. A respiratory therapist might be nearby to do a critical first test, or might need to be called. Once an emergency room nurse was alerted to the possible stroke, he might or might not call the CT scan room, the stroke coordinator, the family, the pharmacy, laboratory, and neurology. And once he was in a room with the patient, he would most likely be leaving several times to get the correct forms, the correct vial to capture blood for four necessary tests and to make sure the family had time to visit. Each nurse had a unique working style. To get to reliable performance with no unnecessary waiting, stroke care needed standard work.

Everyone practices a little standard work in his or her life. Most people put their toothbrush back in the same place every time—the same for coffee in a canister or silverware in a drawer—simply because nobody wants to hunt for often-used items every time. Standard work means identifying common tasks, deciding on the most efficient and effective way to perform them, choosing who should do the task at what time, and having everyone take the same action, the same way, every time. Then, when problems develop, the standard work sequence can be investigated for error and changes can be made to prevent future errors instead of hunting down an individual and assigning blame.

One-piece flow is another concept from manufacturing that saves time. It refers to how a product, or in this case a patient, should move through a process—in one continuous flow, without waiting or warehousing between steps, only being touched to create value.

In a lean environment, employees seek to touch a product or patient once and be done. Get it right the first time, every time. Likewise, a patient should not be parked in corridors or have blood drawn repeatedly for individual tests or have procedures stopped and restarted. And specimens should be sent to the laboratory as testing is needed, as opposed to allowing large batches to accumulate for the convenience of the phlebotomist.

Sometimes, it is difficult for medical staff to see how their hard work might be bad for a patient, slowing the patient's time through diagnosis to treatment. To illustrate the work sequence of a nurse, for instance, the team used a lean tool called a spaghetti diagram. Over a layout drawing of the emergency rooms, an improvement team member charted the path a nurse took to perform every work task required. Sure enough, it looked like someone had dropped a bowl of noodles on the floor and then maybe slipped in the mess (*#3 Motion*).

The team also created a big circle on one wall. Around the edge they wrote the name of each person or department that needed to be in communication on a stroke patient, including neurology, laboratory, pharmacy, CT Scanning, MRI, floor staff, the charge nurse, emergency medical services, neurology nursing, special medical equipment, etc. Then, based on interviews with staff, someone drew a line between the names to show who typically called whom and how many times. At the end, there was a nearly solid circle of crossed lines (*#6 Overprocessing*).

In those crossed and chaotic lines of the communications circle and the spaghetti diagram, the team could see the sometimes-frantic energy that greeted stroke victims.

Coordinating Care

Using a value-stream map that showed each task to be accomplished along the path through diagnosis and treatment, the team redesigned work roles and tasks. Now, a "Code Stroke" call goes to a communications center—usually while the patient is en route to Theda Clark—which sends out a public-address notification and individual alerts to every player. Because there were almost always two nurses involved in the early stage of care—who sometimes miscommunicated or replicated work due to the lack of clearly defined roles—the team assigned one nurse to be the *doer* and one to be *recorder*.

In this way, standard work could be written for each role. The doer starts the IV, hooks monitors to the patient, ensures that blood is drawn and tubes are properly labeled. The recorder asks questions of the patient and family, interfaces with doctors, and records information in the chart.

The team created a Code Stroke book as a single binder with all the necessary forms. When alerted to a stroke en route, a nurse picks up the book and the tubes required for standard stroke lab tests. Posted in the Code Stroke book is the standard work for stroke care—a step-by-step description of the necessary work, in the correct order.

The new book and job descriptions were created to ensure patients got into the CT scan as quickly as possible. Then the team realized that reading the CT scan was treated as a single task, while there were two distinctly time-sensitive pieces of news that came from the reading. First, neurologists needed to know if there was blood pooling in the brain, indicating a hemorrhagic stroke, or if there was instead a blocked artery indicating an ischemic stroke. If it was ischemic, neurologists needed to know where the blockage was.

Getting that first piece of information broadcast is critical in cases like Lee Parker's because it helped determine that she was eligible for the clot-busting drug, tPA. If her stroke had been hemorrhagic, the same drug that ultimately saved her could have been fatal.

Results

The new "Code Stroke" process went live on July 17, 2009, with these results through the end of 2009:

- *Strokes confirmed*: 36

- *Door to CT scan guideline < 25 minutes*: 51% before improvement, 89% after

- *Door to CT read guideline < 45 minutes*: 36% before improvement, 89% after

- *Door to tPA guideline < 60 minutes*: 14% before improvement, 50% after

- *Mortality*: 7.6%[20]

(See Figure 4, Code Stroke Process Flow, in the Appendix.)

After Theda Clark was designated as a "center of excellence" in stroke care in 2006 and all ThedaCare stroke patients were directed there, this facility has had a 60% rise in stroke patients—from less than 200 a year in 2005 to more than 300 in 2009. Improving the process means the Stroke Center is now improving the outcomes and recovery expectations for hundreds of people every year.

As a result of her stroke, Lee Parker had to learn to take naps. She became more conscientious about diet and exercise. But she did not have to relearn a grandchild's name or spend months painfully regaining the ability to walk. Time was on her side.

---

20. Mortality rate by stroke type: ischemic 1.7%, subarachnoid hemorrhage 1.5%, intracerebral hemorrhage 4.1%.

About three months after her stroke, though, Lee was invited to a dinner meeting of ThedaCare's stroke survivors group. After a lifetime of being active in community groups, hospital auxiliaries and the like, she and her husband, John, naturally thought they would get involved. As Lee looked around the dinner tables filled with young and old stroke survivors, what had happened to her really sunk in.

"There were so many people in wheelchairs and using walkers, having real difficulty doing the simplest things," Lee said. "I walked out of that dinner with guilt to my eyeballs. How was I so lucky?"

Time is brain. Waiting is waste.

The Doctor Will Be with You Soon

People are accustomed to waiting for healthcare. For weeks or months before an appointment, in outer offices and lounges on the day of the appointment, patients wait. People grumble about it and are sometimes even outraged by it. But mostly they are resigned to the unavoidable hassle of seeing a doctor (#2 Waiting).

Even before ThedaCare began adopting lean philosophies, leadership decided it could no longer accept the status quo. Fast access to care-givers was quickly becoming a point of competition and delays were impeding good care. "Advanced Access" projects started up throughout ThedaCare's 20 primary care clinics in 2001 to eliminate backlogs and find new ways to see patients immediately.

By 2007, patients at the family practice group in Kimberly, WI, for instance, could consistently get a same-day appointment if needed. Schedulers set aside about 30% of each doctor's day for last-minute appointments—a little more in flu season—and that time was always filled.[21] Once in the door, however, the average stay in the waiting

21. Each of the four doctors at Kimberly has a patient panel of about 2,500 and they see each patients approximately 2.5 times a year.

room was 15 to 20 minutes and there were too many logjams in the daily flow. Also, patients were driving miles to appear at the office, have blood drawn, and then drive back across the same miles a few days later to get results and see the doctor (*#4 Transportation*).

In early 2008, ThedaCare's lean facilitators and an improvement team—including the clinic's doctors and staff—gathered data on workloads, conducted time studies and discovered a few things about the practice at Kimberly that changed their working lives. What they discovered also turned around the fortunes of this small clinic.

The Kimberly Clinic is what you might call a mature practice. The four doctors have been practicing for enough years to each have a loyal following and the majority of patients are over 45 years old. Despite the full patient loads, the practice was losing a modest amount of money every year. About 10% of the patient population had chronic issues associated with obesity and/or heart disease, and that 10% consumed 60-70% of available appointments.

Chronic disease management is time consuming but there is a set pattern to appointments and patient needs. If correctly anticipated, these can be handled without a lot of hand-offs, delays and consultations, saving time for patients and saving costs for the providers. Better chronic disease management meant that the general practitioners at Kimberly would need standard work to treat routine cases more efficiently and effectively.

Over the course of 2008, improvement teams met for week-long Rapid Improvement Events several times to study the issues, make immediate changes, and study the process again. Teams discovered that medical assistants—the skilled helpers who perform initial interviews, arrange lab tests, and take vital statistics—were often the key to a day's work flow. One doctor moved quickly and was sometimes stalled, waiting for his assistant to catch up. Another medical assistant was sometimes without anything to do, waiting for another doctor's slower pace. The old one-on-one strategy of pairing one doctor with one assistant was not working.

Doctors were also frustrated at the amount of unfinished work at the end of a day. Each of them usually had a backlog of electronic records waiting with open questions about prescription refills, drug side effects and the like. The end of the office day for everyone else often signaled the beginning of "chart-time" for doctors. The improvement teams investigated every corner of the business.

The danger with a simple summary of improvements is that this can make a lot of hard-won changes look easy. Some were relatively easy; some were not. It was all worth it, however, given the way a patient's experience changed after 18 months of lean improvements.

When a patient calls today for an appointment, the first question is still, "Would you like an appointment today?" On average, 30% say "yes." Now, a representative leads the patient through a series of questions pertaining to needs, and notes everything in an electronic medical record. In the case of a patient being seen regularly to manage a chronic illness, the medical chart will already have advance notes about what the patient will likely need, and the representative can schedule accordingly.

About 24 hours before the appointment, for the 70% of patients who have made an appointment in advance, staff at Kimberly go through each chart, looking for what tests will most likely be needed. If a chronic disease patient is involved, for instance, staff checks that goals for weight, blood pressure or cholesterol levels are highlighted for the doctor and patient to discuss.

An innovative and somewhat miraculous improvement is evident on appointment day for anyone needing laboratory results. Instead of coming in to the clinic 24 hours before an appointment to give blood or other fluids, which are then taken to a central lab for processing, patients visiting Kimberly get same-day—same-hour—results for common tests, thanks to a one-woman, on-site lab that can handle all routine tests.

To create this high-volume mini-lab, a team mocked up a one-person laboratory and devised more efficient methods for performing certain tests. Teams mapped new ways to simultaneously conduct multiple tests with different timing requirements on limited equipment. Then, they wrote and rewrote standard work so that any trained lab technician could do the work consistently.

The staff at Kimberly is very proud of that lab and often coaxes "their" lab tech, Jenny Ball, out to meet visitors. The physicians always describe Jenny as a treasured asset. Here is why: when a patient needing urinalysis, hematology, or one of seven different kinds of blood chemistry tests comes in for an appointment, the patient gives a sample and then meets with the doctor. Within 15 minutes, the lab results are slid under the exam room door for doctor and patient to review together.

It is true that the new lab needed a few square feet to operate. So, in a 2008 redesign, the clinic eliminated most of the main waiting room. Medical assistants now invite patients back to begin their exam shortly after they arrive. Time spent in the waiting room averages five minutes and 75-80% of the time, the doctor arrives in the examining room within five minutes of the patient being seated by the medical assistant. Every patient leaves with a plan of care that lists what medications have been changed or stopped, time of next appointment, if necessary, and any follow-up actions required.

Waiting wastes not only time, it wastes money. Defects like ordering the wrong tests; needless motions like a nurse wandering the halls looking for supplies; unnecessary transportation such as taking routine lab samples to a distant location; overproduction, as in scheduling more patients than can be seen in an hour; overprocessing by passing patient files back and forth to answer predictable questions; unnecessary inventory, such as expired medications or lab supplies; and the waste of talent that is a highly trained doctor sitting in a room, waiting for staff to send him a patient—all are a waste of money. Eliminating these wastes, and treating more patients without increasing staff effort, has meant a steady rise in revenue. In 2006, Kimberly Clinic lost a typical $400,000. In 2009, for the first time, the clinic turned a profit.

Other treatment groups in the ThedaCare system saw what the Kimberly Clinic was doing and adopted many of the new methods. The full complement of techniques pioneered at Kimberly is being introduced in every primary care practice across ThedaCare.

The Stroke Center learned from Code STEMI work in cardiology. Other primary-care clinics are learning from work done at Kimberly. None of the ThedaCare treatment groups took on the new ways, however, without first conducting their own rapid improvement weeks and learning to make continuous improvement a part of their organization's DNA.

ThedaCare is committed not just to better healthcare and lower costs. The staff is committed to continuous improvement as a way of doing business and a reflection of our organizational identity. In the next chapter, the people of ThedaCare who have gone through the transformation will tell you why.

Chapter 5

Continuous Improvement

The tension had been building all that Tuesday afternoon. The improvement team was supposed to limit itself to working on communication flow, but there were a dozen team members in Labor & Delivery picking through everything that happened between the moment a baby was born and the new family left the hospital. They kept finding issues in the discharge process. Staff members on the unit felt increasingly challenged.

In the middle of it all was a young woman, the mother of a toddler whose serious medical condition had been missed by a ThedaCare team after birth. She had written an angry letter, spelling out exactly how staff had failed her and the boy. In response, she was invited to help fix the process and she joined the team. She was articulate, generous with her ideas, and well connected to a network of other young mothers whose opinion she regularly sought throughout the week. In other words, she was a gold mine of customer feedback and the 12-member team—including then-CEO John Toussaint—was anxious to tackle every issue.

She told the team that nurses kept running in and out of the room during birth, creating a sense of chaos instead of joy. A good fix for that would be stocking all supplies and drugs in the room, which would mean modifying the physical layout of the delivery rooms. The team was up to the challenge. Too much information came at the new mother all at once? The team wanted to write new standard work, breaking up the nurses' instruction on feeding, diaper-changing, etc., into manageable chunks. The team reviewed how doctors performed the baby's first physical, how hospital staff communicated with the new baby's doctor, and whether nurses should accompany new mothers to their cars, to instruct on proper placement of a car seat.

"Enough." The obstetrician's voice was taut as she cornered MaryJeanne Schaffmeyer, then-manager of the obstetrics unit at Appleton Medical Center, that afternoon. The team stopped talking, alert now to the confrontation. "I think we're making too big of a deal out of this one case."

The young mother, still struggling with the repercussions of her son's condition, walked across the room and with a voice full of emotion said, "It's not just about my son. This is about how we work with all children."

For a tense second, everyone waited. Then the doctor visibly softened and the team got back to work. After all, they only had one week to complete the project.

Pulling It Together

Focus on the patient, value, and time. The way that these interconnecting principles lead to rational systems with less waste is so sensible it can seem simple or inevitable. But then comes a critical, foundational element of lean healthcare: continuous improvement.

Over the past few years, several hundred people have toured ThedaCare hospitals and clinics, hoping to replicate ThedaCare's improvement in patient outcomes, staff engagement, and reduced costs. Visitors see evidence-driven improvements, a more scientific approach to healthcare delivery, and lights are ignited in their eyes.

Then the tour guide gets to the part where revolutionary change is required to create a lean organization, and how continuous improvement must be practiced every single day. Suddenly the light in visitors' eyes starts to dim. These are smart people who know enough not to ask for a silver bullet. But they still want one. What ThedaCare has discovered, however, is that a bunch of villagers with sharp sticks (i.e. improvement teams) are far superior to any silver bullet.

Prior Bullets

In the years before lean healthcare, ThedaCare enjoyed the attention of many reputable consulting firms. Each had a program that would address wasted time, poorly deployed resources, and the calcified build-up of faulty communication that everyone agreed was unhealthy.

One firm took two years to help redesign ThedaCare's management reporting structure. An entire layer of management was removed, saving $1 million, and decision-making was pushed to the front-line nurses. All of this was great in theory. But supervisors went from managing 30 people to 120. Nurses were not properly trained or supported in their new decision-making duties and having one-hour meetings once a week to discuss their issues did not resolve the structural difficulties.

A second consulting group spent more than a year teaching employees the "90-day workout," using a rapid improvement approach pioneered by GE. While people began to see that improvement could happen rapidly through concentrated effort, the method was frustratingly laborious and reliant on consultant time and support. Staff could not do the work fast enough to make a real difference.

Another group brought Six Sigma, and after conducting a thorough analysis of radiology, revealed there was a 300% variation in process results. This was shocking until staff realized that most processes had a 300% variation in results. Dramatic variations in performance may seem surprising, but this is more the norm than the exception in American healthcare, where scientific methods have not been used in organizing work sequences. Many processes coalesce organically, without rigorous thought, and are left that way for years, unexamined. So defects per million opportunities fluctuate in the hundreds or thousands. Meanwhile, those who manufacture widgets have closely studied work processes to achieve better productivity while striving for Six Sigma, equaling 3.4 defects per million opportunities, or even perfection.

Measuring processes and pinpointing variation with a Six Sigma program seemed like a good start toward improvement until it became apparent—in the weekly follow-up meetings—that nobody knew how to redesign the work sequences and that ThedaCare, in general, lacked the discipline to stick to a redesign anyway.

In the end, we saw the enemy of our improvement efforts and it was us. ThedaCare's leadership was treating each improvement initiative as a time-limited, finite project conducted by a few members of staff or consultants. Improvements ended when the project was over because nobody was in charge of sustaining change and measuring results. Meanwhile, doctors were still firefighting throughout their workdays and then attending weekly follow-up meetings for improvement initiatives that were in terminal condition. Frustration invaded every building.

In order to change outcomes, leaders at ThedaCare needed to change their expectations and level of engagement. As we began the push toward becoming a lean organization, we understood this imperfectly.

Back to the Villagers

Looking back at the best of the failed improvement programs, there are two repeating themes: empowering staff—the doctors, nurses, and managers actually doing the work—and measuring results. Without a method, these necessary attributes are nearly impossible to hard-wire into the daily work habits of staff. Continuous improvement is that method.

There are two primary mechanisms at ThedaCare for continuous improvement: the team-driven, week-long Rapid Improvement Event and the more narrowly focused PDSA (plan, do, study, act) problem-solving cycle. While there are many additional improvement activities employed at ThedaCare—from identifying patient value streams to redesigning entire hospital units and establishing visual controls—let's examine the core mechanisms first.

ThedaCare's Rapid Improvement Events are team projects. The action of an RIE reaches its peak during one week in which a cross-functional team studies a problem and makes immediate changes to the process. The full event, however, is a seven-week cycle. Prior to the team week, a manager in the targeted area and the project sponsor establish quality, productivity, and throughput goals, pick a team, collect existing data, and conduct new time studies.

Teams usually have a dozen or so members, drawn from front-line staff such as doctors, nurses, and clerks, plus support staff such as pharmacists, radiology and EMS technicians, and others who work nearby, or in upstream or downstream procedures, plus an outsider. The outsider might be from a different department or hospital, or from an outside organization. Teams also try to include patients whenever possible, to ensure everyone stays patient focused.

Day one of the RIE week includes a brief orientation period, with training in lean tools and principles, and details of the project at hand. The team then goes to the department or clinic area, maps the existing state of the process in question, and conducts time studies as staff members work through their usual routines. On the second day, the team develops maps and timelines describing the current and ideal states. From this, members design the future state—taking into account practical realities while improving the process. The goal is always to pursue the ideal state, while improving what can be improved immediately. If machinery needs to be moved or roles need to change, team members often spend part of the day hauling equipment and briefing staff in the area. The difficulty of coming to consensus and then making real changes in areas where habits may be deeply entrenched has led teams to dub this Prozac Tuesday.

By day three, the team watches and assists as those doing the actual work in the target area test-run the new process. By day four, team members write and implement new standard work for the process. Day five, the team reports on early results during a company-wide, Friday morning report-out meeting that includes up to six presenting teams and more than a hundred people in a local junior college auditorium. The report-out is part teaching session, part evangelical lean revival. As senior leaders, we make it a point to attend as often as possible.

Quick Shot

PDSA stands for plan, do, study, act. This is a formatted cycle for thinking about and working through a problem. It comes from work originally popularized by W. Edwards Deming and widely embraced in Japan during the postwar years. Deming, who is often referred to as the father of the quality revolution, believed that improvement must be a continuous loop of activity.

In the first step—*planning*—a problem is identified and studied. This is where data collection on critical processes is especially important, so that anyone starting a PDSA can examine performance of a process over time. Staff members doing a PDSA project are also expected to solicit the opinions and expertise of others in the work area, and add that to the collected data to create informed theories about problems and solutions.

Then there is *do*, or fixing the problem. This means taking action, not writing reports or seeking permission.

Next, the revised process is *studied*, with close attention paid to whether changes in the process achieve the stated goals and is manageable by people in the area.

If deemed successful, *act* is writing new standard work to cement the improvement in place and start planning for another improvement. If unsuccessful, act means returning to the planning phase to seek a new approach to the problem.

At ThedaCare, PDSA has become shorthand for personal development. Because PDSAs are often narrower projects than rapid improvement weeks, each one can be the responsibility of a single person. As areas of the organization become more experienced with lean, staff members are expected to complete a number of PDSAs annually.

In Action

To see how people are using team weeks and PDSAs, let's look at the ThedaCare laboratories—although not as a shining example of how to perfectly execute lean thinking. They are not. What has happened in the ThedaCare labs, however, is a fair demonstration of how ThedaCare's people have seized the ideas of lean and used team projects—RIEs—and PDSAs to create better work environments.

ThedaCare labs employ about 180 people in three locations, with the largest facility traditionally attached to Theda Clark in Neenah. For years, even the simplest testing was shipped mostly to Neenah and processed in big batches. Some level loading among the three facilities early in the lean transformation corrected this to a degree, but it was still a centralized operation until ideas like the single-technician lab at Kimberly Clinic started changing perceptions.

Let's begin further back, however, in 2003 just as lean ideas were rolling out across ThedaCare and laboratory leaders were recognizing they had a crisis in the phlebotomy group. Phlebotomists are the front-line collectors of blood samples for testing and in 2003, nurses were mostly responsible for drawing blood and collecting other specimens. That meant, between changing sheets, administering medications, helping patients to the bathroom and giving information to family members, the nurse was asked to carefully insert a needle into a vein, draw blood, put it in the correct tube for the correct test—there are dozens of possibilities—and affix the right label. Considering the nurses' distraction and workload, it is remarkable that the average was just 941 defects per million samples.

Let's make that math personal. With ThedaCare labs processing about 10,000 blood draws per month, there were nine or 10 mistakes. Nine or 10 times per month, a sample arrived at the lab without a label, or bearing the name of the wrong patient, or the blood of the wrong patient, or had incorrect patient identification numbers on a blood bank tube, causing delay in treatment or misdiagnosis. It was unacceptable.

Leadership stepped in first, deploying a team of dedicated phlebotomists to do all patient blood draws in ThedaCare hospitals. With laboratory personnel now having complete ownership of the process, from blood draw to test results, improvement projects were more straightforward and RIEs began in earnest.

Armed with a few hours lean training and guided by a consultant, teams studied how patients were identified, how samples were collected and labeled and transported—eventually scrutinizing every step in the process. Over the next two years, the process changed radically. Phlebotomists now ask each patient a standard series of questions to verify identity. Every phlebotomist carries a portable bar-code reader to identify the patient from the admissions bracelet and to verify which laboratory tests had been ordered by the doctor.

Within 24 months, the defect rate in this area was reduced to about 250 per million, from 941 per million. That was about the time improvement teams started learning about value-stream mapping to look at the bigger picture and hunt down new areas to improve. By the end of 2007, phlebotomy defects were running at 224 per million opportunities.

Quickly, the RIE work spread to other areas in the lab. In cytology—the study of cells—Pap smears comprise about 90% of the workload and only 69% of Pap smears were being processed in a day. Lab employees were accustomed to thinking of newly arrived samples as *tomorrow's work*. Both ThedaCare-owned and independent clinics were complaining that turnaround on Pap results was too slow, yet lab technicians felt they were working as fast as they could.

Clients were also complaining that the costs were too high. Specifically, clinics were pressuring ThedaCare to drop the cost of Pap smears to match competition from two low-cost mega labs. With 50% of the business coming from non-ThedaCare clinics, the ThedaCare labs were in danger of losing half the business. A team trained in lean principles took a close look at the Pap smear work sequence and knew what had to be done.

Processing a Pap smear can be broken into three parts: registration, slide preparation, and reading. Traditionally, a cytology assistant picked up a sample, entered all the information from the vial's label into a computer, and checked medical histories for prior instance of cervical cancer or unusual Pap smear results. Then, the assistant picked up another vial, registered that one, and then registered another. With a batch of samples registered, she proceeded to slide preparation: placing the vial and a glass slide into an instrument and waiting while the instrument processed the sample to produce a smear that could be analyzed for results. Typically, cytology registered a large batch of vials one day and did slide prep the next. It was classic batch manufacturing—a way to organize work that seems logical but causes delay and inventory buildup while increasing the chance of replicating errors.

In the RIE team's initial time studies, members noticed that registration took almost exactly as long as slide preparation. That meant a technician could begin the slide preparation process, then turn and register another sample while the slide prep instrument was running the first slide. This was one-piece flow, a processing method that assists technicians in catching errors before a whole batch of slides has been mishandled, and which helps everyone keep track of what tubes and slides have been through which processes. Without the wasted time of waiting while the instrument processed the slide, technicians were soon achieving same-day results on Pap smears 92% of the time. Cytologists went from being rushed and always behind in their work to moving through their samples at a steady, manageable pace—with time to spare.

"Team members came to me after we were done and said, 'What do we do with this extra time we've got now at the end of the day?'" said Bill Boyd, who was then the laboratory's business unit manager. "I just smiled. What a great problem."

Even though customers were also demanding new, more expensive imaging technology be added to Pap smear testing, ThedaCare's main lab was able to reduce staffing by 30% at constant volume—through attrition and redeployment of one cytologist to another part of the lab—and reduce the price of a Pap smear by 20%. The Lab's margin took a small hit, but the customers were happy with the faster turnaround time, lower price, and advanced technology, and lean made it possible.

The Power of One or Two

Meanwhile, phlebotomy was dealing with two reoccurring issues in 2007: a slowdown in process improvements and low morale. After more than two years of major changes, phlebotomists on the front lines felt they were not in control of their own world. They moved through patient rooms with trays of needles and tubes to collect samples from people who were almost never happy to see them. Then RIE teams came in, timed everything with stopwatches, and made changes. Phlebotomists were stressed and disconnected from the real work of the hospital: making people better.

In 2007, laboratory leadership began emphasizing daily improvement work in the lab, starting with phlebotomy. The idea was that phlebotomists needed a method for making immediate, finer-tuned changes to their processes, so PDSA became part of standard work. Every morning, phlebotomists who were not out on the hospital floors would meet, review data from the day and week before, and ask what happened yesterday and how could it be improved. From these questions, ideas bloomed and, guided by the teaching of Deming, the staff searched for root causes, designed countermeasures, and took action.

For example, one project was sparked by the lab's ongoing battle with mislabeled specimen tubes. Staff members were always collecting data around the mislabeling issue and found that bad labels sometimes occurred because the portable bar-code reader failed to "see" the black and white code on a patient's bracelet. When this happened, the phlebotomist had to enter a patient record number manually, increasing the possibility of error. Working with a PDSA form that guides the user through analysis and the search for root cause, the phlebotomists found that sometimes the patient bracelets were unreadable because they were badly printed. Or the printer was loaded incorrectly, causing the bar code to print on top of the holes used to attach the bracelet. Or part of the bar code was covered with tape.

Not everything could be solved in a day, but with a list of issues to work on, phlebotomists could use their spare time to work with nurses on how those bracelets were constructed and attached onto patients, or how patient identification was printed. Instead of passing each other anonymously in the halls, the phlebotomists and nurses were now working on common causes, one small improvement at a time. After each improvement was made, it was tracked carefully for 30 days to make sure the new improved method was used and useful.

In this way, phlebotomists have chipped away at errors, cutting the defect rate by another 60%. At the end of 2009, the error rate was consistently hovering around 100 errors for every million opportunities —nearly a 90% reduction from ThedaCare's historic levels.

"What was really cool to see was our team members bringing out defects in the process as they found them," Bill Boyd said.

Results

Staff in the core lab—including clinical pathology and phlebotomy—closely follow the rate of corrected lab results as an overall quality metric. A corrected lab result occurs when a lab error is written into a patient's electronic medical record and then must be corrected. Putting bad results into a patient's record, of course, creates a higher risk of bad diagnosis while the erroneous results are on file. Since launching the PDSA routine in June 2007, corrected lab results have been reduced by 73%.

Speed is another critical factor in hundreds of lab tests. Since reporting on the time it takes to perform each test would be overly burdensome and create data avalanches, lab managers selected three common types of tests to use as proxies. These three tests take different pathways through the lab and so are used as performance indicators for all tests following the same path.

1. The Basic Metabolic Panel, a serum analysis, is a panel of eight tests ordered for about half of all patients admitted to the hospitals. In 2005, 90% were completed in 33 minutes. By year-end 2009, 90% of tests were done in 23 minutes.

2. Automated Blood Count, a whole blood analysis, is a basic screening and diagnosis test with a wide variety of uses and is ordered for about half of all patients admitted to the hospitals. In 2005, 90% were completed in 11 minutes and, by the end of 2009, 90% were done in 9.5 minutes.

3. Troponin, using serum or whole blood, indicates whether the patient has suffered a heart attack. Testing volume is lower, but timing is critical for these tests. In 2005, 90% of tests were completed in 40 minutes; at the end of 2009, 90% were done in 30 minutes.

Abbreviating time in the first two tests means there is more capacity in the lab for additional tests, so ThedaCare hospitals can grow without straining the lab or spending money to expand capacity. The third test is critical for individual patients—who must await results of this test before receiving potentially life-saving treatment.

Productivity in the laboratory overall, as measured by units of output per shift divided by full-time-equivalent employees, rose over these four years (2005–2009) by 24%.

And in Obstetrics, where a young mother helped us see Labor & Delivery from the families' point of view, patient rooms have been redesigned to include locking cabinets and drawers with all the drugs and supplies that are needed for birth. Nurses do far less hunting and gathering. Staff makes an appointment for the baby's first check up and sends all records to the doctor's office before mother and child check out. Instead of lining up a bunch of babies in the nursery and giving them physicals, conveyor-belt style, physicians now do baby's first physical in the patient room, allowing another opportunity for parents to ask questions or report abnormalities. This last improvement probably would have changed the medical outcome for our team member's son. If she had just a little extra time with the doctor, she would have had time to ask why the boy had not passed an important milestone and the boy's condition would have been diagnosed more quickly. He would not have been perfect, but the boy—if diagnosed earlier—would have been better.

The obstetrics team in that initial RIE week identified 140 steps in the discharge value stream. By the end of that week, half of those steps had been removed—many of them involving nurses fetching supplies or babies being transferred to other rooms for tests. The average birth at a ThedaCare hospital is now a calmer and more predictable event. And isn't that what every parent wants?

Setting Priorities

Over the years, those of us leading ThedaCare's lean transformation have also found ways to make those "Prozac Tuesday" confrontations during rapid improvement weeks less likely and less disruptive—if not entirely eliminated.

When the doctor in Labor & Delivery approached MaryJeanne Schaffmeyer to say she thought the team was "making too big of a deal" out of one sick baby, she was really saying that she and the obstetrics staff were alarmed that the team seemed intent on changing *everything*. The improvement team had certainly exceeded its original scope. But under this problem was a deeper one still: identifying a purpose.

Why was the team doing this work in Labor & Delivery? What was the larger purpose and how did it fit into ThedaCare's plans for the whole organization? Nobody knew. In the absence of a clear plan or roadmap, doubt creeps in. And doubt can easily lead to the kind of anxiety that derails a team and a lean initiative.

In 2005, ThedaCare leaders recognized we had a problem with purpose and focus. To highlight the problem, we gathered ThedaCare's leadership in a conference room and had everyone write down each of their improvement projects and new initiatives on a sticky note. Value-stream improvements, marketing campaigns, new human resources, and information technology programs were written on square sticky notes and stuck to the wall. This wall was at least 25 feet long and eight or nine feet high and, by the time we were finished, it was completely covered in paper.

The moment that the exercise was finished, and all leaders had taken in the blizzard of projects that defined our working lives, the problem was obvious. We had too many programs and not enough resources to complete everything effectively.

We needed a method to focus energies on the key priorities and we found it in *hoshin kanri*. Like continuous improvement, hoshin kanri is an essential technique to carry out a lean transformation and it is the last such technique we will cover in this book.

The Power of Hoshin Kanri

Developed in a few major Japanese companies during the quality movement of the 1950s, hoshin kanri, also known as strategy deployment, is a discipline used to focus the work of senior executives. In the United States, it has been deployed by lean executives in many industries when they saw initial enthusiastic organizations fail to become lean, even when everyone's eyes were opened to waste in the processes and the power of lean improvements. This was because leaders had rushed off in different directions, pursuing different ideas of the most important problems to solve. The impact was often too diffuse to hit the bottom line and soon the lean initiative looked like nothing more than frantic action without direction.

At ThedaCare, we used hoshin kanri to identify our key objectives and clearly de-select others in order to focus our purpose. (*See sample diagram used in hoshin kanri in the Appendix, Figure 5.*) Identifying key objectives came out of repeatedly asking, "What is most important?" and "How do we measure that?" More specifically: "What are the most important problems and opportunities for ThedaCare? How do we measure the success of our initiatives for solving problems and seizing opportunities?"

The use of hoshin kaanri, which links our highest-level, "true north" objectives of safety/quality, customer satisfaction, and financial stewardship to specific initiatives, helped keep senior leaders focused on priorities, data, and outcomes, and it's a great tool. But we also needed an enhanced version of the PDSA—known as an A3—to help us take action on strategic issues and to solve problems at the executive level. Bearing the European name for standard 11-by-17-inch paper, A3 is a tool developed at Toyota to lead people through the scientific method of studying an issue, getting to the root cause, proposing countermeasures, and implementing changes. It is designed to fit on a single sheet of A3 paper, to avoid long report writing.

The A3 is useful because it requires managers to define the problem and do a root-cause analysis before launching any type of action. We modified it slightly during hoshin kanri sessions to help executives work through issues in strategy deployment.

On a sheet of A3 paper, a team fills in the following information regarding a significant problem or opportunity:

1. *Title*—names the problem, issue, or topic

2. *Owner/Date*—identifies who owns the problem or issue and the date of the latest revision

3. *Background*—states why the issue is important along with any relevant background information and notes what has been observed at the gemba[22]

4. *Current Conditions*—illustrates the current state of the process in question using pictures, graphs, and data

5. *Goals/Targets*—describes the expected results of improvement and the key measures of success (safety, quality, people, delivery, cost, etc.)

6. *Analysis*—states the root cause(s), and expected progress toward solving the problem

---

22. Gemba is Japanese for "workplace" or, more specifically, it means the place where real value is created in an organization.

7. *Countermeasures*—lists proposed actions, plus a statement as to how those actions will address the root cause and what the new standard work might be

8. *Implementation*—explains what will be done, by whom and when; including a list of performance indicators to show progress, and a training plan

9. *Follow Up*—states anticipated issues in implementation, plus a plan to capture and share the lessons learned from the work and a method to continuously improve or begin the cycle again.

Using this more detailed PDSA worksheet, which puts every problem or opportunity in an organizational context, senior leaders could fully explore root causes, possible actions, and the effects of those actions on the organization before implementing possibly disruptive policies. (*See Figure 6, PDSA A3 Template, in the Appendix.*) And it allowed us to keep asking in a very focused way, "What is important?"

We asked the question repeatedly over six years, sometimes arriving at different answers and always striving to determine the most important needs of the entire organization. As we narrowed down the list of critical needs, we winnowed our major projects each year down to three or four initiatives that could be accomplished in a reasonable time frame and easily explained to the entire organization.

Looking back over our hoshin kanri work, we can see now that we made the error of confining this conversation to senior executives. It is difficult to break the cycle of a hierarchy, even after your eyes are open to the problem. In a more fully realized lean healthcare organization, everyone from top surgeons to freshly graduated nurses, senior adminstrators, and housekeepers should have a voice in defining the most critical work to undertake.

You Are What You Measure

The discipline of hoshin kanri also helped us focus on the four points of ThedaCare's true north: Customer Satisfaction, Safety/Quality, People, and Financial Stewardship. For each of these points, we selected metrics to track our progress toward goals. As the needs of the organization changed—and as our understanding of lean healthcare deepened—the metrics changed, too.

For instance, everybody knows money is important, even for a nonprofit. So, if keeping a healthy income is a critical need of the organization, how does that get measured? Meeting an annual budget is an easy, common answer to how finances are measured. But every budget is a moving target, and budgets are more often a reflection of wishes and predictions than of reality. It would be too easy to claim that financial goals have been met, by virtue of a carefully manipulated budget.

At ThedaCare, we settled on productivity gains as a key sign of improving fiscal health. If employees are using—and wasting—fewer resources every year in the course of their jobs, the organization is moving in the right direction. If more patients can receive high-quality healthcare while ThedaCare has the same number of employees, it is a sign of good financial stewardship. Therefore, productivity is a component of every improvement project, and is the focus of one major initiative each year. As evidence that that productivity was the right metric, ThedaCare enjoyed a dramatic profitability improvement after choosing to track productivity rather than adherence to a budget.

Quality is another critical component of a healthy hospital, one that is difficult to measure because there are so many facets to the idea of quality. An executive team originally tried to establish a goal that would put ThedaCare in the company of the best hospitals nationwide, saying ThedaCare's goal was to be in the 95th percentile of quality rankings nationally. That sounded good, but after discussing the issue, we saw that this goal could still leave ThedaCare's patients vulnerable to a lot of defects and potential harm. (We have shown examples of work in Code STEMI and the Stroke Center where ThedaCare was already at the top of national benchmarks but made the decision to improve its quality dramatically.) Comparative measures simply do not inspire people toward perfection. ThedaCare leaders instead settled on a quality metric of removing 50% of defects every year instead. That means, year in and year out, ThedaCare aims to cut in half the number of defects from the year before, marching onward toward perfection.

In this way, through trial and error and long discussions around the hoshin kanri A3s, ThedaCare's leaders steered toward true north metrics —the few, critical measures to guide everyone in the organization toward the same purpose and ideal. Leaders still rethink these metrics, and nobody believes the current true north metrics will remain fixed forever. As the environment changes, who we are as an organization and what we measure will need to adjust. It is a dynamic world and, as hockey legend Wayne Gretzky said, you have to skate where the puck is going to be, not where it's been.

Sustaining the Results

The biggest challenge in any lean environment can be summed up in a single phrase: sustaining the gain. If, for instance, the discharge process in obstetrics was not written into standard work and people stopped paying attention to the process, there is little doubt that some doctors would revert to lining up new babies in a nursery and giving a first physical there. It's quicker for the doctor and it seems logical —unless you happen to be the parent anxious to ask one last question, or the nurse who is fetching babies and lining them up for the doctor's convenience.

So, how does an organization keep everyone doing the right thing? Three years after beginning the lean journey, we discovered a horrible truth about this issue that had some members of the executive team ready to quit—quit lean, quit trying to improve, and quit ThedaCare.

We were frustrated because the transformation seemed to stalling or rolling backward in some areas. Sustaining the gain was a constant struggle and it did not seem to matter that our staff knew the lean tools and were pressing forward with RIEs and PDSAs.

Finally, some brave soul said to a senior executive, "How are we supposed to change when you keep managing the same way?"

The truth can be a sharp sting.

We were demanding change of everyone while we, the senior leadership, remained unchanged. We were leading ThedaCare the way we had been taught that real business people lead. We were hierarchical and autocratic, keeping a tight grip on all the cards.

To achieve a truly lean environment, however—to sustain the improved processes and keep everyone focused on continuous improvement—*everyone* must change. Lean cannot be delegated to a few. It is a discipline that requires a new way of seeing by everyone in every role and the cultural transformation required is the focus of the next section.

Part II

Lean Healthcare
People

If you are now trying to figure out how to impose the techniques of lean healthcare upon your own organization, stop. Imposing new methods does not work. We spent years trying to force change on doctors and nurses, coax new behaviors, demand different working styles. This did little more than raise everyone's level of frustration.

In the past few years, however, ThedaCare has been undergoing a revolution. After mastering many techniques of lean, people throughout the organization have begun making a profound shift toward becoming lean in their thinking. This was only possible, we believe, through coming to a deeper understanding of the meaning of respect.

Respect seems intuitive, but it is a complex idea, especially in the workplace. As a leader, to have respect for staff usually means giving lip service to peoples' concerns, to say that you hold them all in high regard. This is often a polite lie.

Respect actually means wanting everyone on staff to have meaningful lives, and working actively toward their fulfillment. This is such a critical element of a lean healthcare organization that we have made it a foundational principle. In many ways, it is inseparable from continuous improvement, even though it is distinctly different.

People are not very different in their basic needs. Everyone wants to feel needed, to be an integral part of a team doing good work. Respect for people means helping everyone become integral to the larger team, to find fulfillment in their work through empowerment. By empowerment, we mean giving people the tools to become problem-solvers and then creating the working conditions that applaud solving problems instead of sweeping them under the rug. Without a continuous-improvement environment, people become frustrated because they do not have the tools or the permission to fix problems. A lean healthcare organization trains people in problem-solving, then respects their opinions and experience enough to let them take the lead on improvement.

In this way, you can see how respect for people and continuous improvement intertwine to form the bedrock foundation of lean healthcare. This has been an evolving idea and, in many ways, this second section is about ThedaCare stumbling toward a better under-standing of respect. As leaders, we are still grappling with the deeper meaning, but we do know one thing that you will also discover: change must begin at the top.

Chapter 6

Leadership in the
Lean Environment

U pon his death in 1966 at age 90, Alfred P. Sloan, Jr. was eulogized in the *New York Times* as the dominant force in 20th Century American business. Mr. Sloan built General Motors from a dysfunctional collection of automobile and parts manufacturers into the biggest car company and the world's largest manufacturing company for more than 70 years running. Said Roy Abernathy, president of the American Motors Corporation, in an obituary: Sloan was "the most advanced practitioner of modern management of our time."

Mr. Sloan could not get a job at ThedaCare today.

The problem was his management style. Taught as gospel in preeminent business schools around the world, some of which bear his name,[23] Sloan's methods relied on financial statistics to judge business results, emphasized hierarchy with grants of authority to the manager of each unit of the business, and created the multidivisional "M form" structure.

---

23. Besides the Sloan School of Management at the Massachusetts Institute of Technology, there is the Sloan Master's Program at Stanford in California and Sloan Masters at the London Business School.

The M form, in which dedicated business units such as Chevrolet or Saginaw Steering were judged by their own return on investment and given "goals" (expected results) by corporate staff, eventually caused serious problems.

Sloan was a shrewd judge of managers and was able to put the right individual in the job to achieve the expected results and improve the business. After his departure, however, less-capable leaders defaulted to simply "managing by the numbers." Instead of improving the process that produced the results, business units began to manage the numbers instead, in an endless contest with the finance staff at headquarters. This led to factionalism and a focus on short-term profits instead of long-term value. Much has been written about the folly of using financial equations to drive decision-making, but it is the legacy handed down from Sloan in the form of modern management that has proved the single biggest impediment to lean healthcare.

The traditional organization chart, showing who has authority over what activities, was once celebrated as a triumph of rational thought. But we now know that it has two major flaws: the rigid grouping of people vertically by function and the hierarchical, top-down command structure.

Apples with Oranges

It has been common sense to group all the sales people under one department and to do likewise with accounting, operations, and customer service. The modern management wisdom is that people with similar jobs need to interact easily. So companies set aside offices—or floors or entire buildings—for separate functions such as accounting or operations. This is working in silos—side-by-side with functional colleagues, but in isolation from the rest of the organization.

The problem with this structure is that it focuses vertically on the needs of the departments and their employees, instead of looking horizontally at the needs of the customer or patient. What a customer needs is for the salespeople, contract writers, builders, and technicians across a company to be working in unison to deliver the value they promise. Customers do not want the sales force sequestered off somewhere, talking to each other about clever ways to sell. Instead, customers need salespeople to be thoroughly familiar with the product and the company policies. Likewise, a patient wants a seamless care experience, with a team of knowledgeable people caring for him and treating his disease or injury from start to finish, instead of being handed off between caregivers in different—and sometimes rival—camps.

Using this logic, lean management emphasizes creating cross-functional teams that are gathered around a product—or, in the case of healthcare, around a patient's condition or journey through the hospital or medical office. The patient becomes the organizing focus.

When a company structure is viewed through the lens of this more collaborative, team-driven style, the hierarchy of Sloan's organizational chart—in which the boss bosses and everyone else obeys—suddenly appears unworkable. And yet, the vertical org chart is so embedded in the American idea of how business is conducted that it is very difficult to replace.

After all, think about those who are drawn to top management jobs. They tend to see themselves as born leaders with superior judgment and management skills. In healthcare, many of those leaders are also medical doctors, who have been trained to be firmly autocratic. Once all those leaders are clustered at the top in positions of authority, getting them off their hierarchy is a true challenge.

The Limits of Leaders

In 2004, ThedaCare had a hard lesson to learn about hierarchy. While many lean efforts were underway (admittedly centered on doing rapid improvement weeks and not necessarily on identifying and the most important issues in the organization), one medical-surgical unit had four wrong-site surgeries in the space of eight weeks. Because the unit was not yet engaged in lean work—there were no metrics defined, no focused data collection, and no improvement teams investigating processes—the defects slipped under the radar and the surgical team simply did not report the problem. Even after the third, then the fourth horrible wrong-site surgery error, everyone simply kept quiet.

Thanks to the peer-review process, errors like this do come out eventually. At 10 o'clock one morning, Kathryn Correia, president of ThedaCare Hospitals, was informed of the string of wrong-site surgeries. She verified the data and then immediately shut down the unit's surgical suites. By noon, the doctors assembled for an emotional meeting. Petite and crisply articulate, Correia stood in front of the room of surgeons and explained that the surgical suites could not be reopened until they had a plan to ensure the safety of every patient. Voices were raised and it took a moment for Correia to realize that the surgeons were angry *with her*. She was blowing it all out of proportion, they said. She stood her ground.

Let's leave Correia there for a moment, standing alone in front of a room of angry surgeons. It is a good illustration of one problem with hierarchy that can be called, "It's lonely at the top." Autocratic decision-making means that each executive talks down from a lonely perch. In a collaborative environment, the president of ThedaCare's hospitals would have been part of a team that included doctors from the surgical units, executives, nurses, and others whose only focus would have been fixing the broken process. Instead, on that day, there was a lot of angry blame throwing at Correia.

The surgeons who argued with Correia about shutting down the surgical suites did finally agree on a plan to have an independent auditor present for every surgery to lead the "time out." This was a call-and-response triple check between surgeons, nurses, and the auditor that the right patient was on the table in the right position for the right procedure. It was a temporary, necessary fix for a broken process. Since that time, improvement teams have investigated and improved many aspects of surgical processes to improve patient safety. And random audits of surgical procedures are ongoing. However, looking back, it is easy to see how ThedaCare's culture at that time was not only putting patients at risk, it was hurting doctors and staff, too. There was no upside to reporting error in our shame-and-blame culture and so most opportunities for learning and improvement were lost.

Shame and blame is common to most healthcare organizations. If a nurse or doctor makes a mistake or does not conform to an established standard—and not necessarily a written standard—the repercussions are entirely personal. Here is a typical example: A few years ago, a new surgeon at ThedaCare was singled out as "inadequate" after one of his patients developed a postoperative infection. This particular surgeon was under special scrutiny as a recent hire, so a mistake was considered evidence of deficiency. Once the facts were gathered, however, staff discovered that most of the other surgeons in this unit also had patients with recent infections. An improvement team was able to change certain surgical procedures and establish a containment process, including new hand-washing techniques—which, incidentally, the new surgeon had advocated when he first arrived on the unit.

The new surgeon was exonerated by the data—which proved that the process was more at fault than the individual. But the exoneration came only after emotional trauma and damage to his reputation. It would have been a good lesson in the limits of leadership without good data, and of the blindness that envelops most top-down, autocratic management systems, if the unit and top management had been prepared to hear it.

Going to the Gemba

It was 2006 and about three years into ThedaCare's lean work—always taking a few steps forward and a few steps back—that the lean initiative hit a wall. Lean behaviors were being unevenly adopted and some areas remained obstinately untouched. Morale was dropping throughout the organization. Finally, at the urging of a lean consultant, senior leadership began "going to the gemba" every week. (*See Figure 7, Results of the ThedaCare Employee Satisfaction Survey, in the Appendix.*)

Gemba is another useful word from the Japanese. Literally translated as "workplace," gemba refers to the place where real value is created in an organization. Senior leadership of most companies spend shockingly little time there. If the CEO does appear in the intensive care unit or a busy emergency room, it's usually a backslapping tour, meant to underline his authority and spread the idea that he both cares about and keeps a close eye on operations. At Toyota, on the other hand, going to the gemba meant assisting operations: looking for problems or improvement opportunities and finding out what workers need to stay on target. It means getting to know, first hand, the issues facing front-line workers and helping to work out solutions. It means learning, not teaching and telling.

When ThedaCare's 10 senior executives first started a weekly gemba visit in 2006, we immediately saw a disconnect between our decisions and the reality of front-line staff. For instance, we had recently denied a purchasing request from a clinic for a piece of scanning software related to electronic medical charts. It was unimportant, we said, and too costly. On a gemba visit to this office, however, we observed one administrative assistant repeating the same mind-numbing task over and over. She spent 90% of her day manually entering information into the medical records system that could have been accomplished in less than half the time with—it now seemed—a relatively inexpensive bit of software.

It was a quick lesson in the arrogance of senior leadership. Through our control of the purse strings, we set priorities for our operations in ignorance. We were demanding results when we were oblivious to issues with the processes delivering those results. We didn't know what we didn't know.

Forming Opinions

An important issue we quickly discovered during our gemba walks was that many ThedaCare employees had not yet been properly introduced to lean thinking. Many people had heard rumors that "lean was mean" and involved stopwatches and scrutiny. Too few had experienced the satisfaction of making over their unit to better serve their colleagues and patients.

Internal surveys showed that employee satisfaction—which ThedaCare has always closely monitored—rose significantly after an employee had participated on three rapid improvement teams. ThedaCare was running five or six rapid improvement events every week and including new people every time. But three years in, only one-fifth of employees had been on even one improvement team.

So, Roger and his staff in the Organizational Development office devised a one-day lean seminar for all 5,500 employees. Working in small groups, facilitators introduced lean ideas, had everyone play a game to simulate one-piece flow, and talked about ThedaCare's plans for the future. In surveys taken before and after the seminar, there was some positive shift toward lean. Managers, however, nodded and smiled and went right back to the same old autocratic behavior.

To be fair, the leadership team had not told managers exactly how or what to change—largely because we were still trying to define that, ourselves. But we knew that an essential change in management style at all levels of the organization would be critical to avoid the backsliding that plagues most organizations trying to become lean.

The Mirror

In 2006, senior leadership retreated into an intensive, two-day session in which the questions were: What is a lean leader? How can each of us become a lean leader?

We thought deeply about how to define and encourage a new type of leadership and listed the habits lean leaders would need to adopt. These were focused on seven essential areas: safety, responsibility, improvement, unity, customer-focus, teaching, and respect.

- *Safety* meant knowing the potential safety issues in the unit being managed and ensuring that, if safety were compromised, work would be stopped immediately until the issue was resolved. Safety always comes first.

- *Responsibility* meant effective communication in the manager's business unit, making certain that staff knew what is expected, and that they followed standard work.

- *Improvement* meant using and supporting all improvement tools, especially PDSA, as well as keeping track of relevant metrics and sharing those with the team.

- *Unity* meant knowing ThedaCare's common system-wide measures, asking for help when needed, and anticipating the impact of actions on team members.

- *Customer-focus* meant anticipating patient/customer needs, asking customers if expectations are being met, and designing business models to meet customer demand rather than the needs of the organization.

- *Teaching* meant celebrating success and acknowledging failure as opportunities to learn. This required coaching and willingness to be coached, recognizing what motivates people, while forgiving staff that made mistakes.

- *Respect* meant candor. A lean leader should have regular and honest communication with others, be open to new information, actively seek clarifying data, and develop common understanding with colleagues on issues, particularly those running across the organization.

Versions of this behavioral inventory have appeared in PowerPoint presentations and it is a useful list to have when talking about modeling new conduct. But the list alone has not changed anything or anyone. To create new mangers, we needed to change the job instead of trying to alter the person.

Standard Work for Leaders

Transitioning from autocratic to collaborative management requires full engagement in the lean work. That means using the tools consistently and embracing the discipline of lean—and in particular, standard work. On the front lines where value is actually created, standard work is the step-by-step work sequence required to successfully complete a job.

In a lean factory, standard work is a list of the steps required, in the right sequence—often with illustrations rather than words—the appropriate machine settings, the time expected to complete each work element, and the correct tools to use. Standard work for the recording nurse in ThedaClark's stroke center includes noting in the patient's file each action taken, interfacing with the doctor, collecting specific information from the family, and giving information to the pharmacy.

But how does any of this translate to the job of a vice president of hospital operations? Initially, our executives and managers did not think standard work would apply. Like doctors, they were each accustomed to doing tasks their own way and putting out fires when events went wrong, as they often did. That meant every day was different and every leader needed to be available for the inevitable, immediate emergency. How do you write standard work for that?

Besides, a good manager needs to keep his finger on the pulse of operations, guiding many different areas or functions to work together for a common goal. This means an executive needs flexibility. Is there such a thing as standardized flexibility?

The Management Skunk Works

There was so much resistance to the idea of standard work for managers that testing it out became a kind of skunk works[24] project, quietly carried out by Kathryn Correia and her direct report, Kim Barnas, who was vice president of operations for the Hospitals Division of ThedaCare.

---

24. "Skunk works" usually refers to a secret lab or facility where innovators work. The term emerged from the secret Lockheed factory in Mojave, CA, where aircraft like the U2 and SR-71 were designed and built.

Barnas became an early lean advocate after she used PSDA and RIEs to remake the work of an oncology unit as it prepared to install a robotic radiosurgery system. Called a CyberKnife, the system used radiation beams at high intensity to shrink tumors hiding in the brain or tucked up next to the heart. At $2.4 million to buy the equipment and finish the room, it was a big investment that would give the hospital a distinct competitive edge while giving patients a less-invasive, highly effective treatment option.

What Barnas did not like was the manufacturer's strong recommendation that she hire five new people, including nurses and a physicist, to run the device—a major long-term expense. So Barnas pulled in some lean experts and sponsored improvement teams, which created a value-stream map of a patient's journey through radiation treatment, from first consultation to first treatment. Over the year that the CyberKnife room was being prepared, oncology hosted an improvement team every six weeks.

Every person's job was examined from the patient's point of view and tasks that did not serve the patient were eliminated. Patient-focused care, in this case, meant being extremely time sensitive, as no cancer patient wants to wait weeks for required radiation therapy. Teams worked hard to remove all unnecessary actions that clogged staff schedules and created patient backlogs. In the end, waiting time from first appoint to first treatment was reduced from 26 days to six days.

"We were able to significantly collapse the time between consultation and treatment, which was great," Barnas said. "And in the end, with the waste we removed, we only had to hire two people. Everyone else we got by freeing up existing employees."

Now a true believer, Barnas was already thinking about how to engage independent-minded physicians as lean team players, having lost two radiation oncologists in the move to lean after they decided that a team environment was not right for them. So when Correia asked her to think about standard work for leaders in hospital operations Barnas was ready for the challenge. She agreed that managers needed to change, but did not want anyone handcuffed with inflexible rules. Also, she needed to take into account the very different standard work needs for front-line supervisors, mid-level managers, and vice presidents.

Learning from Tchotchkes

With a team of six people, Barnas observed managers in their leadership positions, mapped schedules, and talked about needs—what the leaders needed and then what subordinates needed from leaders. They began to see that every leader—supervisor, manager, or vice president—was part of an interlocking system, much like the Russian nesting dolls, the tchotchkes, on Barnas' office shelf. Each doll was independently itself, but configured with others to create a greater whole.

This idea is reflected in the standard work now introduced in hospital operations at ThedaCare, which governs 75% of a front-line supervisor's workday, 50% of a manager's time, and about 25% of the time for a vice-president. All leaders adhere to one basic rule: 8 to 10 a.m. is a no-meeting zone. This is when everyone reviews data from the previous day or week and conducts needs assessments for their areas. Then leaders meet in a huddle with staff, following a standard agenda that prompts everyone to think ahead, together, about the risks, quality concerns, and cost issues that might occur that day. From there, top priorities for the day are defined, with an emphasis on intercepting issues before they balloon into problems or crises. Following the huddle, there is time for individual coaching, additional gemba visits, and reviews of important metrics. (*Samples of the standard work for leaders at different levels are included in the Appendix, Figures 8–9.*)

In order to keep everyone's eye on the metrics, Barnas' team also developed a scorecard for each unit, listing the important data for that unit and showing how it affects ThedaCare's true north metrics: customer service, safety/quality, people, and financial stewardship. Once a month, data is collected from all unit scorecards and rolled up into the vice president's scorecard. That "roll up" is done in a meeting where all units are represented, results are reported, and process-related countermeasures are developed and agreed upon if the unit is not achieving its target.

The simple arithmetic of five supervisors reporting to one manager, and seven to 10 managers reporting to a vice president, means that managers at each level must spread themselves between their subordinate teams. Barnas has seven units reporting to her, for instance, and she tries to visit each unit at least once a week. Her standard work, however, is not so rigid that she must visit units in lockstep order.

"If a unit is struggling, I'm there to help them," Barnas said. "And it doesn't mean that unit is doing a bad job. With our standard work routines, nobody is alarmed to see the V.P. on the floor anymore."

This approach to managing work and people is not easy, and not for everyone. Barnas did remove one manager from a business unit who, in all likelihood, would have succeeded in ThedaCare's old management style. While well intentioned, this manager could not make the transition to lean in a way that inspired people to follow.

The Standard Work Proxy

Matt Furlan, ThedaCare's chief operations officer, has three vice presidents reporting to him, all of whom are developing standard work for themselves. In addition to coaching and supervising executives, Furlan is also working to spread standard work on medical procedures across units. For instance, when a team in a surgical unit focuses on reducing infection from catheters, tests the new methods, and gets stellar results, team members write it up as standard work. Furlan then helps to spread the benefits of that work so that better results can be enjoyed across all surgical units at ThedaCare.

Spreading standard work to his job has been trickier. "I'm not even close to where I want to be," he said. "So far, my calendar is my proxy for standard work. I need to work on three different value streams every week with the right people, and I need to dedicate a certain amount of time to coaching, and to being at gemba. So that gets written into my calendar in red and it can't be touched." (*See Figure 10, Standard Work Sample Schedule, in the Appendix.*)

Next up, Correia will be trying to wrestle her own job into the discipline of standard work. "I have no idea what it will look like," she said with a laugh. "But I'm excited about the idea of opening up a set amount of my time to innovation."

Looking Ahead

It is too early in many of our experiments to declare victory, but it is encouraging that standard work for supervisors, managers, and executives is pushing everyone to think ahead. In those early morning hours, before the buildup of incidents large and small, our leaders are trying to get in front of potential problems before they bloom into error. Setting aside time for foresight is producing positive consequences.

Creating a safer environment for patients and anticipating problems has made our doctors happier, too. Even some who complained that lean was an attempt to foist "cookie cutter" medicine on doctors have come around. But not all. Moving physicians to accept and then thrive within a lean environment has been another long-term project, one that requires its own chapter.

Chapter 7

Engaging Doctors

B y the time lean healthcare arrived at Dr. Joyce Bauer's door in the Kimberly Clinic, it had a mixed reputation. Already, one member of the clinic's tight-knit staff had been moved to a different facility when her job operating the switchboard was deemed unnecessary. It was like losing a family member.

Lean facilitators promised a better experience for patients at Kimberly, and all four doctors were in favor of that. But lean facilitators were trying to implement what they called the "Perfect Patient Experience" with stopwatches and odd ideas. They talked about batches and flow. That might be fine for laboratory work or some clerical work, but Dr. Bauer did not like the idea of it coming between her and her patients.

On the Monday morning of the rapid improvement week that focused on Dr. Bauer's patient flow, the team hung a digital clock and a graph on her door and showed her where to mark down the time she entered the room to see a patient and where to note the time she left.

"I told them I wasn't touching it. My assistant could write it down if she wanted, but I thought it was a waste of my time. I didn't go to medical school to do that," Dr. Bauer said.

The time spent in each appointment would be pivotal, however, to standardizing the process. During pre-event data collection, the improvement team found wide variation in Dr. Bauer's appointment times, compared to her colleagues. One doctor at the Kimberly Clinic gave every patient between eight and 12 minutes, consistently. Dr. Bauer's appointments ranged from eight minutes to 35. But she was happy with her style of practice. She might spend more time in one appointment with a chronic disease patient learning about the source of some emotional troubles, she said, and keep the next exam brief, if possible. Dr. Bauer would often run late, but her patients seemed to understand, even appreciate her willingness to spend extra time with others.

Her days were long but Dr. Bauer, who grew up on a dairy farm an hour's drive from Appleton, developed a system that had worked for her for years. She saw patients all day, one after another; dealt with questions and phone calls at the end of the office day; and then at home, after her two boys were in bed, she finished her notes and closed out the day's medical charts.

On that Monday evening, after being studied by the RIE team all day, Dr. Bauer sat down at home and started a list. She wrote down everything she hated about being measured and judged, and about the recommended changes in her workday for this proposed Perfect Patient Experience. Then she listed a few good points that could come of it. Both she and the clinic staff might be more efficient. She would probably apologize less for lateness. She definitely approved of keeping track of quality measurements and looking for ways to improve. Data would help her—all of them—see what needed changing. Lean seemed to offer better, if not *perfect*, patient outcomes. The "good" list was outweighing the "bad."

"I did a little self-analysis," Dr. Bauer said. "I decided to try and think of Craig Clifford (Kimberly office manager) as a coach instead of a judge. He said that the goal was not to change the doctor, but to change the process of delivering the care. I decided to trust that."

Over the next three days, Dr. Bauer found she could abbreviate appointments by having a medical assistant better prepare each patient and ask more questions—especially about what medications were being taken at what dosage and with what regularity, about which Dr. Bauer is exacting. She learned to ask an assistant for help getting additional information for patients during the appointment, instead of getting it herself later.

In this way, Dr. Bauer was learning to disconnect the primary work —diagnosis—from incidental work such as hunting down files or information. Once the tasks are seen individually and ranked in importance, it is far easier for a physician to choose which work to do and which pieces of business to relegate to staff. In manufacturing, this might also be called "load leveling," or spreading tasks out more equitably, so that one person is not overly taxed, bogged down and holding up the entire working group.

Dr. Bauer also learned that "one-piece flow" simply meant doing all the work surrounding a patient's visit in real-time whenever possible, instead of saving her charts to finish up at the end of the day.[25] That meant if an appointment took eight minutes, she had the rest of that allotted time to make follow-up phone calls or finish documenting her notes into the chart.

After the medical assistants were trained to predict questions and treat-ments using standard templates, Dr. Bauer's appointments were reliably shorter and followed a set pattern: 10 minutes for acute visits (colds,

---

25. Dr. Bauer reports that she still takes home about half her charts, but has less work to do on each chart. "We're constantly tweaking the process and changing how we work with the team," she said.

sprains, etc.), 25 minutes for chronic illness like diabetes, and anywhere from 15 to 27 minutes for physicals. Knowing this, the Kimberly staff now sets appointment times more accurately.

By involving the staff more and documenting chart notes during the patient appointment when possible, Dr. Bauer started to understand what Craig Clifford meant by one-piece flow. Batch work was not better or easier, it was just a long-ingrained habit.

Friday came and Dr. Bauer's improvement team joined five other teams, plus an audience of more than 100, in the junior college auditorium where Friday RIE reports are presented for all of ThedaCare. When it was her team's turn, Dr. Bauer took the stage and looked out into the rows of faces. In the style of a penitent at an Alcoholic Anonymous meeting, she said, "My name is Joyce Bauer, a doctor at Kimberly Clinic, and I am a batcher."

The room erupted in laughter and applause. When Dr. Bauer completed her report, a man stood up in the audience and said, "My name is Dr. Mark Hallett and I am a batcher, too."

The Roots of Autocracy

To understand the chasm that lies between most doctors' expectations about medical practice and the type of practice needed for lean health-care, it is helpful to have some sympathy for how doctors are trained. Medical education is still based on an apprenticeship system that goes back to ancient Greece. Young doctors are trained by specialists, who pass along great knowledge in concert with their idiosyncrasies.

Loyalty to one's teacher is highly prized. In fact, the Hippocratic oath does not begin, "First, do no harm," as popularly believed. Those words are not in the oath at all. The first promise is, "To hold him who has taught me this art as equal to my parents and to live my life in partnership with him, and if he is in need of money to give him a share of mine, and to regard his offspring as equal to my brothers in male lineage and to teach them this art—if they desire to learn it— without fee and covenant; to give a share of precepts and oral instruction and all the other learning to my sons and to the sons of him who has instructed me and to pupils who have signed the covenant and have taken the oath according to medical law, but to no one else."[26] Most medical schools have given up the practice of having doctors recite these promises, or use an updated version of the Hippocratic oath, but some sense of this fealty remains and physicians still tend to be more loyal to their specialty and mentors than to their co-workers and hospital.

The men and women who do well in medical school are also perfectionists, great believers in delayed gratification, and are often lacking some essential people skills, says Dr. Hallett, a sports medicine specialist, confessed batcher, and ThedaCare Physician's senior medical director. Long hours and overwork in medical school and residency programs encourage quick, decisive judgments and little collaboration. Psychologists call this a kind of asynchronous development: exercising the logical brain without developing emotional or social intelligence.

"Medical school, residency programs, all of that is like living inside a tube," Hallett says. "We spend our twenties in libraries and hospitals while other people are experimenting with who they are and having fun. Meanwhile, we're breaking all sorts of cultural taboos, like dissecting dead bodies and examining the genitals of strangers.

"Life inside the tube is filled with experiences that are rich and rare— like giving a cardiac massage to a man while another doctor sews up the bullet hole in his heart. In the tube, we don't make any money and most of us rack up a lot of debt, but we're all told that when we get

---

26. Edelstein, Ludwig; Owsei Temkin, C. Lilian Temkin (1987). Owsei Temkin, C. Lilian Temkin. ed. *Ancient Medicine*. Johns Hopkins University Press. p. 6.

out of the tube it will be worth it. So we delay gratification, take pride in our perfectionism, and are encouraged to cover up mistakes for fear of malpractice lawsuits."

Not every doctor would describe medical education as *being in the tube*, but most will describe the same sense of isolation from nonmedical people and pursuits, delayed gratification, and debt. According to the Association of Medical Colleges, 87% of medical school graduates have outstanding loans; 79% of those graduates owe more than $100,000. A lucrative career is a doctor's only avenue to climbing out of that hole.

Admitting Error

In a lean environment, doctors and nurses must allow mistakes to be visible in order to perform root-cause analysis and fix the process. But showing mistakes hits most medical providers in a vulnerable place —right in the collective fear of lawsuits and a highly conditioned need to be heroic.

Doctors are deeply reluctant to point out the mistakes of others, much less officially reprimand one another—knowing that they all hide mistakes, and being sympathetic to the pressures faced by colleagues. To issue an official reprimand is to risk destroying the career of a doctor. So errors are not discussed, except in the rumor mill. (We will discuss ways to eradicate the most common form of reprimand, shame and blame, in the next chapter.)

Moving doctors from their hard-earned autocracy into becoming team players, where they share responsibility and—to some degree— decision-making is no simple matter. As ThedaCare's lean initiative spread across hospitals and clinics, leaders of the movement made mistakes and learned a few lessons worth sharing that can be summed up in three words: data, urgency, and trust.

Data Drives the Scientist

Deep within every doctor, a scientist lurks. Trained in data collection and usage, taught to rely on the scientific method, doctors are most comfortable with arguments that include numbers. Unfortunately, the fear of malpractice and damaged reputations has made medical professionals profoundly reluctant to publicly release scores on critical quality markers. That fear must be conquered.

A lean healthcare initiative always begins with data collection and dissemination. What data is collected, and how it is presented, will change over time as an organization's needs and focus changes, but getting and broadcasting the facts is always necessary because data can cause people to change behavior.

For instance, shortly after that early improvement week in Labor & Delivery—when a young mother helped redesign the birthing process—a group was taking a closer look at the neonatal value stream and noticed that a surprising percentage of babies were delivered earlier than the normal gestation time of 39 or 40 weeks. Preterm birth is defined as occurring at or before 37 weeks and 12.7% of U.S. babies are born preterm, exposing them to medical complications and developmental delays. However, a number of recent studies have shown that babies born even a bit too early—at 37 or 38 weeks—have a greater chance of chronic respiratory disease and learning disorders than children born at 39 weeks or later.[27] At ThedaCare, 35% of babies were born during this "early term" period.

An improvement team dug deeper into the data, made additional inquiries and found that many of these babies were delivered early on purpose—by inducing labor at a prearranged date agreed on by mother and doctor. It may have been convenient for physicians and

---

27. "Many Women Miscalculate Time to Full-Term Birth," from the website Medline Plus, a service of the U.S. National Library of Medicine and the U.S. Institutes of Health, Nov. 9, 2009, http://www.nlm.nih.gov/medlineplus/news/fullstory_92133.html

families, but it put those babies at higher risk of complications at birth and often resulted in weeks spent in the neonatal ICU. (ThedaCare tracks babies' time spent in the neonatal ICU as one measure of the relative health of premature babies.) The team worked with staff and doctors to create new protocols, including setting a 39-week lower limit for inducing labor.[28]

Adherence to the new protocols was spotty at first. Then, physician performance data was posted on walls in the Obstetrics departments, with every physician's name over his or her track record, meaning no labor was induced prior to 39 weeks gestation for scheduling convenience. There was 100% compliance on the new protocols within a month. As a result, premature babies requiring intensive care now spend an average of 16 days in the ICU instead of the previous 30.

Doctors are competitive by nature. It is a necessary attribute to getting through medical school and then earning desirable residencies and fellowships. Making data public—if the data is honest and relevant—taps into every doctor's competitive nature. Presenting unblinded physician performance like management did in Labor & Delivery caused some grumbling, but it also ignited a drive to be the best.

Data Can (and Should) Drive the Patient

For the public, straightforward comparative data is difficult to acquire. Even simple statistics such as the rate at which patients are infected during a hospital stay can be difficult to find. Disclosure laws vary state by state and even when hospitals are required to report infection rates to an independent oversight organization, the information does not necessarily get reproduced in a public-friendly way. Data can confound as easily as it can inform, after all.

---

28. Cherouny P.H., Federico F.A., Haraden C., Leavitt Gulio S., Resar R., "Idealized Design of Perinatal Care," IHI Innovation Series White Paper, Cambridge, MA, Institute for Healthcare Improvement (2005). Available at www.IHI.org.

Data accessibility needs to change—and become standardized—to give healthcare providers impetus to improve. Currently, hospitals with poor quality records can be financial winners, as long as their performance remains unknown. If people are informed as to the quality and safety records of all hospitals, however, the hospital that focuses on improvement should have the advantage.

In Wisconsin, a diverse group of hospitals, physician groups, and health plans now provide data voluntarily to the Wisconsin Collaborative for Healthcare Quality. The Collaborative includes the largest healthcare systems in the state and makes all information it collects available on an easily searchable website, with quality data available by provider and condition type (www.wchq.org).

A woman with a heart condition who is shopping for a healthcare provider could look at all participating systems in her area for both cost and quality of care, based on standard quality markers. If looking at data from 2007, for instance, she would find that Theda Clark and Appleton medical centers had the best quality/price ratios in the state for congestive heart failure care, but that the higher-cost Gundersen Lutheran Medical Center in Lacrosse had slightly better quality scores (98.5 to Theda Clark's 97.6).[29]

Comparatively Number 1

One important note, as Dr. Hallett points out, is that comparative data is good for the consumer, but not always good for making the lean healthcare argument to physicians. Consider diabetes care. There are three main goals in treating diabetes: controlling blood sugar, blood pressure, and cholesterol. Any member of ThedaCare Physicians[30] could call up the Wisconsin Collaborative's comparative chart for

---

29. http://www.wchq.org/reporting/quadrants.php?category_id=0&topic_id=17&providerType
   =0&region=0&measure_id=22&disclaimer=1
30. The organization of family, internal and pediatric physicians that are employed by ThedaCare.

diabetes care and see that his group was best in the state on keeping patients' sugar, blood pressure, and cholesterol in control. If ThedaCare Physicians is ranked first, why change?

What the chart does not show is that only 25% of ThedaCare's diabetes patients have all three measures in control. Indeed, 75% of patients have one or more measures over the limit, leaving them at increased risk of blindness, limb loss, and death. Knowing this might leave potential patients with a different idea of the quality that those top-ranked physicians are offering.

Therefore, lean healthcare advocates like Dr. Hallett prefer to judge physician performance against perfection (an absolute), instead of against one another (which is to say, relatively). To do this, he and others use defects per million opportunities—like Six Sigma measures in manufacturing. This way, the patient shopping for a doctor could see, for instance, what percentage of diabetes patients were in a safe range on all measures. At last, potential patients could have objective information.

Urgency

If a man is disinclined to swim in a lake, one quick way to make the activity desirable is to set fire to the platform on which he stands. Swimming then becomes not just desirable, but necessary. To get anyone to leave a comfort zone and strike out in new directions, a burning platform is required.

In healthcare, the burning platform can often be defined as provider frustration. Doctors are almost universally aggrieved these days by growing paperwork, longer hours for less money, and patient anger. ThedaCare has had some success identifying that frustration, getting doctors to air their grievances, and then channeling it into improvement activity.

Also: "Never let a good crisis go to waste," to quote Rahm Emanuel, White House chief of staff. The H1N1 swine flu virus was a good opportunity for ThedaCare to create an organization-wide disaster plan. Staff used PDSA cycles to help organize a massive project into manageable pieces, which helped further embed PDSA into the working habits of staff.

Or, for an extreme example of a burning platform for change, let's go to Orthopedics Plus. In 2006, while many doctors were struggling with lean healthcare, the eight independent orthopedic surgeons who comprised the orthopedics practice at Appleton Medical Center packed up their bags and their patients—representing a major chunk of revenue for this hospital—and formed a competing orthopedics surgery across town. It was both a major setback, and a great opportunity.

Using lean tools such as 2P (Process Preparation)[31], a team started from scratch to design a better model for musculoskeletal care. The team wanted a more integrated approach, based on the type of care journey a patient actually takes through orthopedics. So instead of employing eight very expensive and independent surgeons, Orthopedics Plus now employs three surgeons and four primary care/sports medicine doctors who collaborate on the different stages of patient care. Four doctors specializing in rehabilitation—where a patient might spend the bulk of his time on the path to getting better—were moved to Appleton Medical Center from another location so that musculoskeletal care could be concentrated and expertise could be cross-pollinated. The new, more integrated unit was christened Orthopedics Plus and opened for business in 2006, around the same time that the competing private orthopedic surgery opened across town.

---

31. 2P (Process Preparation) is an event in which a cross-functional team investigates a work area, and then reorganizes the physical layout and work sequence to remove waste and create better flow. A 2P is often used when designing a new layout that requires construction.

Dr. Hallett and other designers of the unit—including Jenny Redman-Schell, now vice president of Physician Services and Orthopedics Plus—spent weeks visiting primary care doctors all over town, making a case for the integrated care model. Those referring doctors would be key, they knew, to retaining at least some fraction of orthopedic surgery. But they were up against eight very well-known surgeons.

While the first two years were occasionally rocky, Orthopedics Plus patient satisfaction surveys quickly showed stellar results. Scores were in the 76th percentile nationwide in 2006 and 2007.[32] Appleton's primary care doctors have continued to show a preference for Orthopedics Plus, referring about 80% of all orthopedic patients there.

In the first two years of the new model, Appleton Medical Center was able to retain about 60% of its revenue from orthopedic surgery. The unit's income has now stabilized to the level it was at before the surgeons walked out—although it is expected to exceed the old model—and teams are continuing to ask how this integrated practice can better serve patients.

Trust

Here are a few important, remarkably simple rules for converting physicians into lean healthcare advocates: never lie; be willing to admit management mistakes; ask for opinions and take their advice seriously; be forthright about intentions. Perhaps most important: be clear about the process of care delivery and how it needs to work.

In 2006, around the same time that Appleton's orthopedic surgeons left, morale problems were becoming evident with the majority of physicians. ThedaCare hired a consultant who interviewed physicians over a few months and revealed to management some hard truths.

---

32. The survey was altered after 2007 and comparisons are not available.

First, leaders in the lean transformation had not adequately explained lean healthcare or widely sought physician help with initiatives because it was thought doctors would reject lean as being a "manufacturing thing." Leaders had not made the case for needing change and, without good data for comparison, most doctors thought they were doing fine on quality. Change seemed like a discretionary activity.

Second, focus on the patient had led leadership away from thinking about the healthcare provider as the center of the universe. That was fine in one way, but it meant that leaders had missed an opportunity to apply lean tools to fix the concerns of providers, such as on-time starts for surgery, ease of access to medical records, and accuracy in lab results.

In physician interviews, the consultant did find a deep current of loyalty to John, who was seen as committed to improving quality and burnishing the image of ThedaCare. But doctors were still suspicious of the methods being employed.

In a series of meetings with medical staff following the interviews, 12 physicians committed time to form a special joint committee of the medical staff and the ThedaCare Board of Trustees to identify the most important elements the doctors wanted fixed, and then set out a plan to make it happen. ThedaCare's CEO, hospital president, chief medical officer, and senior executives of marketing and IT were all involved, sending the message that leaders were serious about changing the environment for physicians.

One critical piece of intelligence that came out of the joint committee was that physicians, no matter how committed to quality healthcare and positive change, kept falling back to the same argument against lean: "healthcare cannot be standardized." Doctors feared that lean would institute "cookbook medicine" and force their medical practices into someone else's mold. To counter this, leaders developed the concept of *the middle flow*.

In every healthcare journey, there are three distinct movements: upstream, middle flow, and downstream. Upstream is everything that happens before a doctor sees the patient, from setting appointments to getting vital statistics, laboratory tests, and asking why the patient wishes to see the doctor. These activities directly affect physician effectiveness and can be improved greatly by lean teams. The downstream flow includes getting additional information to the patient, running follow-up tests, dispensing prescriptions, and setting new appointments. Again, all of these activities affect both doctor and patient, and can be improved to increase accuracy, patient satisfaction, and remove waste.

The middle flow, where doctors examine the patient and have a dialogue about care, cannot be standardized. It is not the goal of lean healthcare to make physicians all behave in the exact same way; doctors are not robots.

With the help of an improvement team, Dr. Bauer found some useful tactics to help her middle flow become more effective and predictable, which ultimately helped lighten her workload. But nobody told her what to do and mostly, improvements in the Kimberly Clinic happened to the upstream and downstream flow. Those improvements include the on-site laboratory, enabling physicians to get test results during the patient's appointment. Assistants and nurses, now trained in the protocols of care for chronic disease, are more like team members than order-takers.

It is critical to explain to everyone this concept of the middle flow, before rumors and anxiety have doctors convinced that lean healthcare's goal is to interrupt the relationship between doctor and patient.

"I would never go back to the old way of doing things," Dr. Bauer said, after working one day at a different clinic that had not yet implemented the New Delivery Model (renamed from Perfect Patient

Experience to acknowledge the improvement for doctors and staff, as well). "Working as a team and using standard work is much more effective. Most important, the quality of care is better and the value to the patient is greater."

Bringing Everyone Along

After a critical mass of doctors had moved toward the lean side of the fence, isn't it logical to hope that others would follow? At our most optimistic, leadership hoped that an enthusiasm for lean would sweep through the organization as people saw changes occur that were in the best interests of patients and themselves. However, changing the behaviors of a large, multisite organization requires more than just buy-in from leaders and physicians. As we show in the next chapter, a lean conversion also requires understanding the current culture and creating effective countermeasures.

Chapter **8**

Remodeling Behavior

D
r. Mark Hallett was still learning how to be a physician when
he got a quick lesson in healthcare's disciplinary style. He
was finished with medical school and working through a
general-practice residency in Minnesota when he was offered a shift
moonlighting in the local hospital's inpatient psychiatry unit. Being
broke and heavily in debt, of course, Dr. Hallett gladly accepted.

One evening, Dr. Hallett was on a different floor of the hospital when
he was paged to the psychiatric admitting unit, where a man had
become agitated. Nurses were keeping the man under control and they
needed a doctor to prescribe a tranquilizer. Dr. Hallett started toward
the unit, but was delayed en route and when he arrived in psychiatric
admitting, the man had flown out of control and kicked a nurse in
the groin, rupturing a testicle. The nurse's injured testicle had to be
surgically removed.

The nursing staff made it clear without making a formal complaint
that Dr. Hallett was at fault. They told each other, loud enough to be
overheard, that the doctor should have ordered a sedative, even sight
unseen, for the agitated patient. No doctor or supervisor confronted
Dr. Hallett; he was just never invited back to work in the psychiatric

unit. He was shamed without official reprimand; he was blamed without rigorous inquiry. Shame and blame is so prevalent in the healthcare industry that it is often cited as the underlying culture of hospitals and clinics. And it is one of the largest hurdles to overcome in the journey toward lean healthcare.

Culture Wars

The phrase "corporate culture" has been so overused and abused that it can mean just about anything. In this book, by culture we mean to describe a pattern of behavior that is so widespread and ingrained in a particular group, it is expected and sometimes codified. When people in healthcare talk about the culture of shame and blame, they refer to a common set of expectations in the medical field about how transgressions are—*and are not*—handled. Only recently have people in healthcare started to talk about the damage shame and blame has caused.

As disciplinary models go, shame and blame has a distinct advantage: it's fast and easy. A cursory glance at a situation is all the evidence needed to decide on a culprit. And feeding the rumor mill with the guilty party's name is infinitely easier than launching an investigation and then going through channels to issue an official reprimand. But shame and blame has a terrible price. In that environment, there is no motivation to report errors or safety issues. If staff is blind to error and its cause, there is little hope for improvement.

In the early years of ThedaCare's lean transition, this point was highlighted for John when an introductory Rapid Improvement Event was scheduled on the medical floor of one of the hospitals. The nursing staff invited John to come and talk to them about lean, prelaunch. John did his homework before the talk, looking up the available data for that floor, and found a surprisingly low medication error rate.

After giving an overview of lean thinking and talking a little about the importance of having good data to see the true picture, John asked the assembled nurses to what they attributed their very, very low medication error rate.

A nurse in the back of the room raised her hand. "We don't report errors," she said. A silence fell over the room and every head hung down, waiting for this nurse to be blasted for her admission.

Taken aback, John paused for a moment and then said, "Thank you for being honest."

The room loosened up and slowly, the nurses started to air their grievances. The electronic process for reporting errors was balky and slow. Nurses had to page through several screens and waste precious minutes to report an error, and then there was no upside to honesty—only the possibility of blame and retribution.

Not long ago, another nurse said, someone on that floor had been fired for a medication error. John was shocked and doubtful, as it was not ThedaCare policy to fire people for making mistakes. But listening to the nurses, John realized that it did not matter whether someone had been fired or not. They all believed that a colleague lost her job for making a mistake and that would drive the nurses' behavior until trust could be established.

In fact, after seven years of intensive lean work, examining every aspect of complex processes, ThedaCare has found that individuals are very rarely the cause of a bad outcome. Mistakes are usually the result of a bad process. But if people do not report errors, how can bad processes be fixed?

John promised the nurses that nobody would be fired for reporting a medication error. In fact, it was not policy or practice to fire nurses for such errors, but he could see the nurses needed to feel protected.

He guaranteed them cover. For months, however, error reporting was still uneven. One nurse in the area—a loyal ThedaCare employee with 30 years' experience—ultimately quit and wrote an angry letter upon exiting. She told John that while he talked about improvement, she had to do more with less and her manager was completely uninterested in the problems she tried to address. John had long suspected that the leader in charge of this area had been working at cross-purposes with lean and was too mired in the shame-and-blame mind-set to move forward. The manager said all the right words about error reporting and implementing staff suggestions when talking to leadership, but in one incident after another, staff members were dissuaded from investigating root causes and subjected to the old shame-and-blame rumor mill. Improvement planning in the area met with passive resistance. After many discussions and no positive results, the leader was let go and replaced with an executive who believed that improvement begins with accurate error reporting.

The Culture We Want

ThedaCare's goal is now to have every employee be a problem-solver. Taking personal responsibility to solve problems, and working with others to improve conditions for all, creates an environment of continuous improvement and respect.

To understand the impact of error reporting and personal responsibility, let's look at a common drug error involving the powerful blood thinner, warfarin.[33] Every month, patients at Theda Clark and Appleton medical centers receive about 700 doses of warfarin to treat various issues of the heart and circulatory system. Too much warfarin puts a patient at risk of spontaneous bleeding, bruising, and nosebleeds. Under dosing

---

33. Warfarin is the generic. ThedaCare hospitals use Coumadin for an anti-coagulant, but we have used the generic name here for simplicity.

can cause blood clots. So daily monitoring of a person's blood-clotting capability—with an INR test—is clinically necessary. Managing and monitoring warfarin therapy requires vigilance, and there had been talk about finding better methods to do this. But the issue was brought home in a profound manner in early 2008 when an elderly gentleman fell on his way to the bathroom.

It is an all-too-common event in hospitals everywhere: frail patients attempt that short walk to the bathroom and fall. The underlying problem might be loose cords and tubes trailing on the floor, furniture in the path, failure to wait for the proper assistance and, always, the patient's own infirmity. In this case, the elderly man was dizzy. He fell to the floor, hit his head, suffered a cerebral bleed, and died.

In a shame-and-blame environment, the nurse on duty probably would have been blamed for "letting" the patient walk around. Instead, a team of clinicians led by Richard Berry, Pharmacy clinical operations manager, conducted a root-cause analysis to better understand the incident and identify those factors that may have contributed to the patient's fall.

As Berry discovered, when the man fell his INR was well above therapeutic boundaries. While dizziness from lying in bed and receiving new drugs probably made him fall, the high amount of warfarin likely created or exacerbated the cerebral bleeding. Error-proofing, then, required Berry to understand how this patient's INR rose above the therapeutic range and to make sure it did not happen to others.

Warfarin is a notoriously difficult drug to control. A variety of foods interacts with the drug; it metabolizes differently in nearly every body. There are many different theories on how doctors should administer warfarin therapies. In order to place controls on the work, Berry and his team of colleagues identified a safe range on the INR.

A therapeutic range is between 2 and 3.5. The safe zone was 1.7 to 4.9. Below 1.7, the patient was deemed to be in danger of developing clots; above 4.9 put patients at risk of spontaneous bleeding.[34]

Berry's team first retrieved all INR data and found that 40% of patients receiving warfarin in the two hospitals were testing outside of the safe zone and 17% of the time an INR was not available on the day a warfarin dose was given. The majority of those patients outside the safe zone were testing on the low side and Berry's team found that 30% of warfarin patients with INRs less than 1.7 were being weaned from the drug to regain blood-clotting abilities prior to surgery. Another 70% of patients had just started the drug and it takes most people between three and six days to get into therapeutic range. All of these patients were deemed legitimately subtherapeutic.

The opportunities for improvement were in the 3% of patients testing high, with an INR over 4.9. Also, the team found that 120 doses of warfarin were being administered to patients every month without a current INR.

Working with physicians, the team set about creating evidence-based dosing guidelines for warfarin. There were so many different theories and protocols in place—just about every doctor had his or her own methodology and ingrained beliefs about warfarin, most developed at medical school—that after the team set new warfarin protocols, they needed to ask almost every physician to change. This required newsletter articles and individual and group meetings to introduce doctors to the latest clinical studies and to explain the need for a uniform protocol. Eventually, the new dosage guidelines were adopted throughout the hospitals. In early 2008, 3% of warfarin patients tested high; at year's end, the percentage dropped to one-half of 1%. Next opportunity for improvement: failure to perform INR testing.

34. The average person, who is not in need of warfarin therapy, has an INR reading of one.

When the improvement work began, the prevailing mindset among physicians and pharmacists was that obtaining an INR every 48 or 72 hours was acceptable. The team was faced with deciding on a definition of "current INR" that allowed clinicians to safely manage patients on warfarin therapy. Recent clinical studies have shown that hospitalized patients become far more sensitive to warfarin and really need an INR every 24 hours. Not all doctors believed this, however, and it was doctors who were in charge of ordering INRs, even though it was pharmacists who were tracking the numbers. Again, the team negotiated with physicians and finally decided that pharmacists should be responsible for ordering INRs. Further, the team defined "current INR" as every 24 hours.

To ensure uniform testing, pharmacists built alarms into the electronic medical records of warfarin patients that show when an INR is out of date or out of range. Also, pharmacists pull up a daily report showing all warfarin patients. Next to each name is either a check mark, showing a current INR, or a stop sign. With these controls in place, the hospitals moved from 120 patients per month with out-of-date testing to zero.

Obtaining daily INRs prior to warfarin administration directly resulted in that sixfold improvement in the percentage of patients getting too much warfarin—from 3% to 0.5%. ThedaCare's most fragile patients are now far less vulnerable to serious bleeding consequences, all because an error was reported and a member of the staff asked why it happened.

In the lean organization, employees are empowered to investigate events such as this fall to determine the underlying cause, identify safer practices and prevention techniques. There are hundreds of stories like this at ThedaCare now, adding up to a tidal shift in how employees are perceived and how they perceive their roles. But improvement projects alone cannot do the job of changing the organization-wide behaviors.

Beyond Data

In the same way that processes cannot be improved without data, ThedaCare has discovered that improvement cannot be completely driven by data. This was discovered in an early improvement project in a physicians' group that had a few outmoded, cumbersome processes.

Early in the project week, after timing various processes and mapping activities, a team looked at all the available data and came to this conclusion: the practice did not need a receptionist. In fact, a few work sequences dealing with telephone call routing would be faster and easier without her. The problem was that the receptionist—a loyal employee who had been occupying that or similar positions for 25 years—was on the team. Of course, the receptionist was quickly reassured that she would be redeployed to a new job. But in that moment, after listening to her job being described as unnecessary at best, she did not want to be redeployed. She angrily resigned and across ThedaCare, people began describing lean as mean.

The worst part was that, those who led the improvement project knew beforehand that the receptionist's position was in danger of evaporating. They let the facts speak for themselves instead of preparing people for the possibility. Now, it is part of standard prework for a rapid improvement week to consider the possibility that people might need to be redeployed.

If so, someone from Human Resources meets with the group, talks about job possibilities outside the unit and asks for volunteers. Retraining is now a standardized part of the redeployment package, and Human Resources staff are organized with a reassignment cell that goes to work immediately when there is any hint that improvement activities might result in the elimination of someone's job.

Respect for People

It is a common enough claim: We respect our people. But, do your people know that? Respect is a quality that must be actively injected into organizations. As leaders of a healthcare organization, we need to constantly ask:

- Are our staff and doctors treated with dignity and respect by everyone?

- Do staff and doctors have the training and encouragement to do work that gives their lives meaning?

- Have we recognized staff and doctors for what they do?

Respect is more than just words; it must be embedded in how we work and interact with colleagues and coworkers. Healthcare management is still largely in command-and-control mode. Leaders talk about how to make their wishes—our commands—clear to employees. People do not talk much about how to listen, even though the clearest way to show respect for employees is to ask for their opinions, seek their help in fixing what is wrong, and give them the training to take charge of improving their own work areas.

As ThedaCare has discovered repeatedly, this kind of respect cannot be cultivated overnight. Most hospitals and clinics are firefighting full-time. Employees are running flat out—looking for supplies, recovering from errors, seeking the most basic information—and exhausted when confronted with what seems like an insurmountable array of activities that need to be improved.

Improvement teams need to take the waste out of practices so that front-line staff can stop scrambling long enough to make clear judgments. Then, care providers need time away from their regular jobs to learn about problem-solving and waste reduction and put those skills to use. That means working on improvement teams and learning the PDSA cycle so they can apply it in their own work area.

By working in teams and feeling the immediate effect of waste reduction and more rational processes in patient care, employees learn to trust that "improvement" does not mean "more work" or job losses. Once this threshold is crossed, employees are more willing to offer opinions and suggestions, and put energy into follow-through. Then, with employees fully engaged in the work, woe to the leader that fails to give public recognition to their efforts.

At ThedaCare, recognition might mean regular bratwurst cookouts to celebrate work in the cardiac care unit, or it might mean a big racetrack on the wall of a hospital unit, each racecar bearing an employee's name, to illustrate how many people have implemented improvements using PDSA. The form of recognition is less important than the frequency and the sincerity of appreciation.

Getting Beyond Point A

A culture does not turn on a dime. If the default mode for people at work is negativity, fear of making mistakes, and self-protection, encouraging people to take positive action on their own initiative can be a very hard slog.

When trying to effect real change, it is important to remember that professionals in healthcare have mostly had years of conditioning in the shame and blame environment. Attitudes and expectations cannot be transformed across the board in a week, a month, or even a year. Some individuals will embrace new ways, but it takes time and diligence to alter those ingrained behavioral expectations that we call "culture."

At ThedaCare, the idea of change was well received in the beginning of our efforts, but it became clear pretty quickly that people were humoring leadership during those early "introduction to lean" meetings. There was a lot of nodding and positive murmuring, and then everyone went back to their work areas and did their jobs in exactly the same way as always.

When the message was consistent and insistent enough—and if people saw a way to use the lean initiative to their own benefit—they might step forward to join a team. But even then, most people were not converts. Most of those interested in lean had to work through a few improvement cycles before becoming truly engaged in lean efforts.

Roger, who has spent years studying how people learn and work together in groups—in what he calls "communities of practice"— would eventually describe this as the five stages of change: initiation, reality, resistance, compromise, and integration.

Initiation: the introduction of a new approach to work, in which people begin to recognize its attributes, seek out more information, and get involved in experiments. This stage is about interest, not commitment. People want to know more and find out how the change will affect them personally. Because people are showing energy about the change, this is often mistaken for commitment.

Reality: learning and testing the limits, benefits, and demands of a new approach. This stage is about testing and feedback. It is the scientific method at work, although informally. People ask if the promised benefits are real or not, if there are unknown downsides, and if the program will help or hurt the individual. In this stage, the early adopters discover positive elements to the change and feel validated, while those who are skeptical or resistant find everything that is wrong. Their opposition is often validated at this point.

Resistance: a desire for the perceived comfort of the past or a rebellion against new methods. In this stage, because obstacles to the change are beginning to emerge, people begin to realize that the change will not generate a perfect outcome and will require real effort on their part. Longing for the "old ways" is often coupled with thoughts of rebellion and people may toy with refusing to cooperate, either passively or not.

Compromise: acceptance of limitations and the willingness to consent to uncomfortable change in order to achieve personal and group goals. At this stage, people begin to align with the change—either convinced that the change is good overall, or willing to compromise to make things work. Either way, things can begin to move forward with energy.

Integration: full engagement by working with others to achieve organization-wide goals, reflexively reaching for the tools of the new approach to solve problems, and incorporating personal goals with those of the organization. New behaviors become habits, data trends move in positive directions, and trust in processes grow. (*See Figure 11, Five Stages of Change, in the Appendix.*)

Movement from one stage to another can be wrenching, particularly when change is happening to an entire group. Individuals do not arrive at the same stage simultaneously, and those running ahead or behind can feel pressured to stay with the group. Resentment can easily follow. To make matters worse, if promises are broken or unintended negative consequences occur because of a process transformation, people may actively try to reverse change. This can result in a temporary feeling of distress and chaos, which is a normal part of the change process itself.

The old blame and shame culture is likely to emerge at this point. When people resist change, others tend to blame them for being an obstacle and diminish their role in the new process. Organizations must learn that resistance is a good and necessary part of the process. Without sufficient resistance to test and challenge the new ideas, true buy-in and commitment to the new order will be elusive at best.

One of ThedaCare's oncology groups is a good case in point. The people in this unit were already suffering a good bit of job dissatisfaction, mostly due to shift-scheduling difficulties, when lean was offered as the route to a solution. For years prior to the arrival of lean, employees had a difficult time finding temporary fill-in help for their highly technical jobs. It was just as hard to train an outsider to be a temporary nurse in this unit as it was for everyone else to take on the missing person's extra duties for a shift. This was a mostly acceptable arrangement, so long as only one person was missing. Staff in the unit knew change was needed and, as they learned about the ability of lean to simplify jobs and streamline tasks, it seemed like the answer.

A sense of immediacy took this group through the initiation stage fast. But "interest" is often misdiagnosed as "engagement." This group had not yet fought through the stage of resistance when, in conjunction with an early Rapid Improvement Event, they put together a sub-team to figure out scheduling. The sub-team came back with a schedule that threw everyone into chaos—sparking turf wars in the hallways and on personal Twitter accounts. Resistance was rampant and so ardently expressed that the unit finally became open to management intervention. After a full airing of grievances and fears, the group eventually fell, exhausted, into compromise.

ThedaCare's lean leaders work to help groups avoid full turf wars, of course, but some emotional responses to change are unavoidable. Change can create insecurities in the strongest personalities, and leaders must be prepared to deal with this.

Roger has two rules for working through emotionally charged situations in a group dynamic:

1. *Do not ignore emotional responses.* In fact, seek them out. People confronting change are often fearful or wounded or angry. Let emotions be aired, without giving them too much weight. The emotional statement can contain key information about how to make changes palatable to the group.

2. *Do not be immediately rational in the face of resistance.* Resistance is an emotional response. It must be respected and allowed to air before rational solutions are proposed. Emotion is energy, which is exactly what is needed for engagement. Make a point of listening to the person or group's emotions, give them a framework in which to understand their heated response, and then help turn that emotion toward the creation of solutions and approaches to the problems being expressed. When ready, the members of the group will begin to exercise their rational power for the benefit of change.

This does not mean you need trained therapists on staff. But those who facilitate lean projects must be prepared for emotional outbursts in order to recognize what the group needs.

Dirty Hands

Organizations that use consultants to help launch a lean initiative, as ThedaCare did, will find that many lean consultants adhere to the "learn by doing" ethos. They will insist that the only way to learn lean is to get out to gemba and do kaizen work. Introductory seminars, they say, are a waste of time.

This is called the dirty hands approach and, in the beginning, ThedaCare followed it religiously. It was difficult to get enough employees through the process, however, and many times doctors and nurse practitioners were unwilling to give up a week to be on a team. Still leadership persisted on this path, and kept careful data on how many people had been on a team and thence—leaders hoped— converted to lean.

After about three years, Nancy Gurnee in ThedaCare's Office of Organizational Development did a more thorough analysis, cross- referencing monthly pulse-check surveys on employee satisfaction against lean-team experience. The results, which became the foundation of her master's degree thesis, showed that there was no tipping point of lean-influenced employee engagement until after three events. (*See Figure 12, Employee Engagement Results, in the Appendix.*)

ThedaCare, the largest employer in northeast Wisconsin, has about 5,500 employees at 40 sites, with a 9% turnover rate. Getting each employee onto a rapid improvement team, much less three, has proved impossible even after seven years of nonstop kaizen. Another method had to be found.

Besides launching the one-day seminar, "Learning to See," (*described in Chapter 6*), leadership wanted to become far more deliberate about developing skills. The Rapid Improvement Events could not do all the teaching and training. So, leaders developed a training program with three facets: learning theory in a seminar, receiving personal coaching from a mentor or as part of a team, then practicing those skills on teams or with a PDSA project.

In a manner consistent with what is known about adult learning, ThedaCare's lean training programs focused in a rigorous way on the knowledge, skills, and behavior that individuals require to become successful problem-solvers within a community of professionals. The process is more intensive; it is narrow and deep instead of hoping to provide all employees with brief and shallow exposure.

Despite our consultants' dire predictions, there has been positive movement in employee pulse surveys, even after one "Learning to See" seminar. When asked their opinions on statements such as "I better understand why we must be urgently focused on making improvements," and "I believe ThedaCare is fully committed to improving patient safety," employees were more positive after a seminar. Nearly 29% of people without RIE or seminar experience strongly agreed with the 10 questions, for instance, while 41.3% of people strongly agreed with the statements after attending a seminar.

Another Change Conundrum

In the literature of modern business management, there is great reverence for change agents, nimble companies capable of change, and just about every other kind of change. Change is good. Except, along with change, people require constancy of direction. Organizational systems and methods require consistency and steady direction as well.

At ThedaCare, when it was time for a change at the top, we realized that there were unique challenges to making that change—to maintaining consistent direction within a culture of change. We also knew that most efforts to change organizational methods and culture last only as long as the leadership bringing the changes remains in place. How could we do better?

Chapter 9

Succession

In the middle of 2006, John came to a decision. After six years leading the organization and five years fighting to get lean adopted across ThedaCare hospitals, clinics, and corporate offices, John knew that he was, metaphorically at least, stuck all over with the arrows of long battles with physician groups and staff.

During those six years, ThedaCare had sold off its HMO health plan, lost all of the orthopedic surgeons in one hospital, and seen morale plummet. On the other hand, quality of care was increasing fast in 2006 and attracting notice. Morale was starting to trend upward, but John believed his personal stock had suffered in the early battles.

Also, John had a very good idea of what it took to be a transformational lean leader and what it took to be a steady-state lean manager, moving the organization incrementally but relentlessly ahead. He could recite a list of necessary attributes of a lean manager off the top of his head and he knew those qualities did not describe him.

John was a great communicator and a better instigator. He was good at lighting fires, but he was not the kind of calm and steady facilitator needed to keep the fire burning in the right direction. And he was already looking at a larger playing field, wanting to spread the lean healthcare revolution beyond ThedaCare. It was nearing time to go.

Succession planning, which had always been high on John's agenda, now moved to the top. Preparing for a smooth transition is vital work for any business, but it is critical for lean organizations since so few experienced leaders know lean. At ThedaCare, we spent years building this nascent lean organization and knew that an autocratic outsider with a different agenda could destroy it in minutes. It was still a stretch for some people to take responsibility for their own work environment and it would have been a relief for them to fall back into the old ways, waiting for orders and keeping their heads down. But John was thinking about those at ThedaCare who had eagerly adopted lean, put themselves on the line, and applied their talents toward making real change. This group—growing in number—believed in the power of lean and John could not let them down.

ThedaCare needed to find a lean CEO—someone who embraced the principles and would use them to formulate ThedaCare's strategy. At the time, there were no lean healthcare systems to poach for leadership, but looking at his senior executive team, John counted a number of individuals with enthusiasm and fresh energy. He quietly asked who among these wanted to be CEO and a few hands went up.

This was the beginning of a two-year PDSA cycle focused on succession in which John studied the issue of lean leadership, created individualized training programs, and personally mentored the CEO candidates. He expanded their portfolios and watched them carefully on gemba walks. Due to confidentiality and personnel concerns, we will be vague about the candidates. Still, the experience was instructive and should underline the importance of leadership transitions in a lean environment.

Ultimately, John's goal was to present at least two internal CEO candidates to the board of directors who were well qualified, hungry for the job, and committed to lean. If he failed, his legacy would probably be an almost-lean organization, where the idea of continuous improvement had come briefly to life but then sputtered and died, leaving people reluctant to put energy into the next initiative. If he succeeded, the board would have a wealth of good choices and a leader prepared to advance the lean initiative into its second generation.

Plan: Determining the Attributes of a Lean Leader

There are some traits that all leaders must have: a talent for listening, being heard, and moving others to act; a desire to pull the levers of power; a willingness to step to the front of the crowd. Guiding a lean organization, however, requires that leaders acquire or emphasize additional, seemingly contradictory traits.

Lean executives are, above all, facilitators and mentors. Just consider the gemba walk, where a lean CEO observes work in progress, looking for opportunities to remove waste and help employees produce better products with less effort. A lean CEO uses his or her time at gemba to learn—an innately humble act.

Over time, John developed a list of leadership traits he was seeking. A lean leader must be:

- Patient

- Inquisitive

- Keenly interested in problem-solving

- A good communicator

- A mentor who likes to see people succeed and wants to be in the middle of the action, not stuck behind a desk.

To make the initial leap to a lean organization at ThedaCare, a revolutionary firebrand was needed. But the next phase of the job was to instill lean into the very fiber of the organization. For that, John thought, a deliberate, calm mentor and problem-solver was required.

This is not the standard-model executive being produced by U.S. business schools, much less American medical schools. (*See Chapter 6*.) Nor are leaders necessarily born with lean attributes. John concluded that the truly lean leader must be developed at the gemba.

From the executives who expressed an interest in being CEO, John identified a small number hungry for the job and who would use that passion to keep lean moving forward. Then he devised a plan to mentor each of them to point where they would be prepared to take the helm.

Do: Expanding Candidates' Horizons

Like most large healthcare operations, ThedaCare has a wide diversity of management activities. Overseeing a group of family practice offices emphasizes different skills from those needed by leaders of urban hospitals, hospice services, or emergency response.

Therefore, John first assessed the previous experience of his CEO candidates and gave all of them new jobs, allowing them to acquire experience in different areas of the business. Successful performance and broad experience is always important to a board of directors, as well as to the candidate's understanding of the organization. An important note: This was also a time of heightened sensitivity or anxiety for job candidates. In most large companies, certain areas of the business have more prestige than others, so it was important that it did not appear a CEO candidate was being demoted in the new job assignment.

In late 2006, while John was looking at CEO candidate experience, ThedaCare was also entering into complex and sensitive negotiations with its largest physician group. John assigned the CEO candidates to manage different strategies related to physician relationships, giving each an opportunity to prove to the board that they could successfully deal with ThedaCare's most powerful employee group.

In a lean organization, hoshin kanri offers good leadership opportunities for job candidates to display their leadership abilities among their peers. When deciding who should team-lead the major projects that are selected from a hoshin kanri process, succession and executive training opportunities should always be considered.

Study: Observing the Performance of the Candidates

John also set aside coaching time for each candidate as he or she grappled with their new jobs. He did not tell the candidates this, but the coaching had a dual purpose: help the candidate perform better through feedback, while watching to see how well the candidate reacted to that help.

Over the years of working closely with colleagues in team environments, John had become convinced that a person's willingness to be coached was a fundamental barometer of success. He worked at being a good coach—respectful and helpful without being paternalistic—and noticed that those who responded well also seemed to work well on teams and to get work done. Those who avoided being coached or became defensive seemed to have a set idea of how everything should work—their way. Inflexibility was not a good trait for a lean leader.

Each candidate also received personal instruction on the PDSA cycle and finished projects that proved they could take very complex strategic issues and put in place sustainable improvements. John had the candidates make their reports to the board in person, allowing them to prove they could field tough questions.

Finally, John spent as much time as he could observing the candidates with their subordinates. In a more mature lean organization, this would be easier to accomplish because senior leadership would routinely take gemba walks together and work together on teams. It was good timing that, at ThedaCare, the senior executive team had recently begun weekly gemba visits. This gave John the opportunity to see the CEO candidates engaging in dialogue with subordinates and seeking out opportunities for improvement.

Succession planning also needed to be spread through the organization, John believed, and so he began asking every one of his subordinates, "Who is going to replace you?"

With the CEO candidates and other executives, John worked out plans to increase the skill levels of their subordinates and to set aside time for mentoring their potential successors. As senior leaders began thinking toward the day when they would have standard work, and what that standard work would look like, the leadership team agreed that development of direct reports must be part of every executive's calendar.

Lessons along the Way

For all that went right with John's succession planning, it often felt as if it was teetering on the brink of disaster. The candidates were anxious for the decision to be made; John was still firefighting so much that he did not have all the time he wanted for coaching and mentoring. The secrecy and competition surrounding this specialized mentoring created unavoidable tension. And there was no specific time or place set aside for candidates to train.

ThedaCare desperately needed standard work for succession planning, but leadership did not stop and take the time to create any in advance. If we could start fresh in succession planning methods now, we would create a two-pronged approach.

First, succession planning would be part of every leader's standard work. Mentoring and coaching subordinates to fill bigger shoes would be part of every executive's job description. Looking for potential leaders to train for managerial jobs would be part of every manager's mission. And ThedaCare is working on creating special training in effective coaching methods.

Second, organizations would create standard work for a smooth transition in each senior executive job. If everyone knows what to do to be considered for jobs and knows in advance the steps he or she will need to take to compete for that job, the anxiety of the unknown will be removed from a process that is inherently stressful.

If there had been an implementation plan for the entire organization— an example of which has been developed and is in the next chapter —we would have known to be prepared for pivotal actions such as the training and installation of a new CEO. What is obvious now is that the old Boy Scout credo—*be prepared*—is still an excellent rule.

In the end, John realized that the CEO's most important role is to develop people and in this, he found liberation. He handed off some responsibilities to his potential successors and then mentored them as they worked through problems involved with these responsibilities. John began to enjoy facilitating rather than controlling. Suddenly he had time to remove barriers for the candidates, get them the resources they needed, and highlight their achievements for the board of directors.

Act: Beginning Again

In February 2008, John publicly announced he would be retiring soon as ThedaCare's chief executive officer. He offered the board of trustees his short list of trained replacements and waited for their decision.

In April 2008, ThedaCare's board announced that Dean Gruner, ThedaCare's chief medical officer and senior vice president, was the new CEO. A family physician who had been the chief medical officer of the Touchpoint Health Plan until ThedaCare sold that business, Gruner had served in several leadership positions including senior vice president of physician services. An early adopter of lean, Gruner was described as "uniquely qualified to be president and CEO," by Walter Rugland, chair of the ThedaCare Board of Trustees.

Gruner recently declared ThedaCare's new goal as an organization: to make every employee a problem-solver.

As John left the CEO's chair, he became president of the ThedaCare Center for Healthcare Value. This not-for-profit organization was created by the ThedaCare board to spread the word about lean healthcare and provide resources for the hundreds of hospitals and healthcare organizations that are struggling to reduce waste and increase quality of care using lean healthcare.

If ThedaCare has been working through a massive PDSA cycle as it works toward being lean, the next iteration of that PDSA is taking lean to the entire industry. John is continuing to fight for transparency of performance data, to be made available to all Americans, and working to redesign Medicare and commercial insurance payments to focus on rewarding value.

The work goes on.

Chapter 10

Action Plan

Do you think you can do better? We hope so. For all the work of the last seven years, ThedaCare has still just scratched the surface of lean healthcare's potential.

We welcome competition. In fact, every hospital, physician group, and health plan that joins the lean effort ultimately pushes everyone in healthcare to secure better medical outcomes, lower costs, and better experiences for patients and staff. Someday, the word healthcare will not always be followed by crisis—if we can focus on the patient while creating value (rather than waste) and minimizing time to put healthcare on the mend.

But how and where to begin a lean transformation?

The triumphs and stumbles of ThedaCare's journey toward lean, described in these pages, is not the only template. Lean has been introduced in a growing network of hospitals and implemented in many other industries over the past 30 years with great success when done skillfully. We look to those experiences for guidance, as well.

This much we can say: senior leaders are always the key to making and sustaining a lean transformation. Many times, lean initiatives have begun in middle management with great energy and hope, only to sputter and fail when faced with senior management disinterest or lack of understanding. To make lean successful, there are a few bits of mandatory business that only the most senior management can accomplish. This chapter provides a short list of those tasks.

If ThedaCare were to start a lean initiative again today, we would do a few jobs in a different way and different order. This list does not always reflect what ThedaCare did. Rather it is what we would do today with the benefit of experience.

1. Identify the crisis.

When the platform on which you stand starts to burn, action is the only choice. Senior leaders need to find that sense of urgency by clearly identifing and naming the crisis in order to convince staff that action is the only choice.

Without a burning platform to create clarity and urgency, most people are happy to agree that change is needed—elsewhere. That other department really needs a makeover, right? Without a strong case for change, staff will view incoming ideas as an optional management project and sidestep new responsibilities.

In 1999, Ariens, the snow blower company from Chapter 1, was teetering on the verge of bankruptcy and everyone knew it. As one last-ditch effort before the doors closed forever, management tried lean. From executives to engineers and operators, Ariens employees threw their energy into lean as if their jobs depended on it, which they did. Within two years, the company had become such a success story that we were working on their production line—for a few days, anyway—trying to discover their secret.

At ThedaCare, John identified the burning platform as a quality crisis. But after naming the crisis, he insisted that ThedaCare stop comparing itself to other hospitals—where it looked pretty good—and start using objective measures from manufacturing, such as quality at a Six Sigma level. This was a tough sell. Ultimately, the argument about how to compare quality measures lacked the urgency of the true problem, which was that the quality crisis was resulting in death and injury for patients. Quality of care and slow response times should have been all the urgency ThedaCare needed.

The quality crisis is really the burning platform for all of healthcare, plus the fact that no one—patients, care providers, businesses, or governments—can afford the added cost of waste in the system.

If we had focused clearly from the beginning on quality's effect on patients, doctors and nurses would have been far more likely to join the lean transformation. They did, after all, work hard to join a *helping* profession. The lesson here is to make the burning platform emotional and immediate. For that, quality is your best argument. The bonus is that the steps required to improve quality will also reduce cost.

2. Create a lean promotion office.

Companies have failed in their lean attempts by erroneously deciding that a lean promotion office is a layer of bureaucracy. They have followed misguided advice to "just do it" without any technical assistance to managers. But just going to the gemba and doing kaizen— no matter how exciting—has very limited usefulness and is usually detrimental to an organization's long-term improvement goals.

A lean promotion office is critical for planning and managing change to ensure that employees are educated and involved in lean. A high-level executive should be tapped to lead this office as a full-time job, reporting to the CEO.

At ThedaCare, John selected 12 of his best managers and clinicians to become full-time lean facilitators. These were two-year assignments, after which facilitators were moved back into line management roles. All 12 agreed to the assignment and today most are in key leadership roles with deep-rooted knowledge of lean principles. Today there are more than 35 lean facilitators who are dedicated full-time to lean activity.

An organization committed to lean should aspire to have 3% of the work force assigned as full-time lean facilitators. The goal should be that all managers have at least two years' full-time experience in continuous improvement. We also believe it is imperative to hire deeply knowledgeable teachers or consultants to work with the lean promotion office. In the beginning, we didn't know what we didn't know. So, we also needed to visit other companies, participate on their teams, and learn from other executives experienced in lean.

Next, move all quality functions in your organization into the lean promotion office. Do not divide quality into clinical and administrative issues when you move quality into the lean promotion office. If you do, physicians and nurses may end up seeking other avenues to quality improvement, shattering the organization's focus. Finally, do not allow lean and quality to become divided in the minds of your employees. If this happens, lean will earn a reputation as being about cost cutting alone. Quality and efficiency are inextricably linked in a truly lean organization.

3. Find change agents.

There are agents of change throughout your organization, just waiting to be unveiled. These supervisors and senior managers and front-line caregivers probably do not know yet that they have the capacity to lead major change.

Here is how you will recognize them: They will be complainers and local agitators who hear about lean and seize upon it to make the changes they want. They will be a Jamie Dunham, the nurse who wanted respect and meaningful roles for nurses and ended up helping to create Collaborative Care; or a Kim Barnas, who coveted an expensive new cancer-fighting therapy and helped transform the radiation therapy practice before going on to create standard work for executives. After discovering that lean principles help them solve seemingly intractable problems, agitators become champions and early adopters. These are your change agents. Give them tools and air cover and they will help lean take root in your organization.

Work on solving physician and staff problems first, before attacking more patient-focused issues. This may sound like backward priorities, but this is the way that you will win over the people who will then use lean—repeatedly—to improve patient experiences.

Finally, find change agents on your board of directors. At least one of them will likely be implementing lean in his or her company. Give all board members a chance to champion the changes. Keep them informed of lean's progress and the barriers you find. Put them on kaizen teams. Without the support and assistance of ThedaCare's board of trustees, our lean journey would have completely derailed after three years.

4. Map your value streams.

A value stream is the set of steps that delivers a given type of value to the customer. A value-stream map records all these steps and their current performance. These maps are used to study both individual processes, such as laboratory tests or knee surgery, and larger functions, such as the Human Resources plan for training all employees in lean principles. The goal is to understand the true customer experience and journey— whether it belongs to a patient or employee—from start to finish.

In healthcare, the patient often must make a circuitous and disconnected path through many departments deploying many resources, in order to obtain care. That path becomes clear when you create maps showing all the steps and information flows, for example, for the birthing process or the experience of a heart attack patient from the time an ambulance is called to the time the heart artery is opened up with a balloon. You need to create these maps to see waste of many types and to determine where errors usually occur.

These maps have been an epiphany for doctors and nurses, who see just how difficult a patient's path can be. This discovery usually drives them into action to use lean tools to create easier medical journeys for their patients. So value-stream maps are also a lever to move hearts and minds.

At any one time, between 14 and 16 ThedaCare value streams are being actively mapped and managed for improvement. This means a concentrated application of lean improvement resources to drive significant change, in which the goal is always 50% improvement year over year.

5. Engage senior leaders early in strategy deployment.

Another common mistake of lean initiatives involves outsourcing improvements. There are plenty of consultants who will launch lean with a campaign of kaizen events, explaining that everyone will learn by doing. This leaves senior managers free to (probably) work at cross-purposes to lean. Also, consultants who are not working closely with senior management will not have a plan as to how the improvements all fit together to improve the patient experience, reduce costs, and serve the organization's long-term goals.

Instead, senior managers must be intimately involved in lean through strategy deployment, or hoshin kanri. As described earlier, hoshin kanri is a standardized process to help an organization select and focus on the few key priorities. At ThedaCare, we established true north metrics to keep us focused on the four measures that truly matter. Make no mistake: everyone believes that his or her proposed projects are the most important. So, winnowing down your list of truly critical measures is some of the most difficult work you will undertake.

We spent six years asking the question, "What is most important?" until we all agreed on four things: customer satisfaction, safety/quality, people, and financial stewardship. Knowing the four points of ThedaCare's true north enabled us to define nine simple metrics that kept leadership focused. As ThedaCare's immediate priorities and understanding of the lean journey have changed over the years, the metrics collected have changed as well. There are some common categories, however. When looking at customer satisfaction, ThedaCare typically tracks whether patients have good access to healthcare, turnaround time for lab tests or treatment, and quality of time, which generally refers to the amount of face-time patients have with caregivers. Quality and safety metrics usually track mortality and medication errors. The people section might look at OSHA recordable injuries and HAT[35] scores for staff. Financial stewardship usually focuses on operating margin—or profit—and productivity. (See Figure 13, True North Metrics, in the Appendix.)

Once the true north metrics are agreed upon, make sure that all major improvement initiatives are focused on those metrics, and that every department tracks data that address those metrics. ThedaCare would have made far faster strides in our lean conversion had we begun strategy deployment from the beginning with clear metrics.

---

35. HAT stands for health assessment test, a measure of the health of a person's lifestyle.

6. Acquire and disperse knowledge broadly.

ThedaCare's lean initiative began with the idea that one only learns lean by doing. We agree that there is great value in learning lean by making real improvements. But in ThedaCare's case, strict learn-by-doing meant putting 5,500 people through a week-long Rapid Improvement Event and the logistics soon became insurmountable.

Therefore, large organizations with even a low turnover rate need to combine kaizen-type team weeks with something like hands-on, single-day seminars and internships. ThedaCare's seminars use simulations to present the theory of lean and group discussion on the reasons to pursue lean. It was not intended to be a comprehensive lean training, but by using seminars with simulations, all employees could receive some introduction to lean within three months—enough to understand the essence of ThedaCare's goals and direction.

Learning lean without being on a week-long event is also possible through personal training in the PDSA cycle. All ThedaCare managers are now expected to mentor subordinates through PDSA projects and to ensure that those subordinates, in turn, guide their teams through the same training. In healthcare, this is probably easier than in other industries because PDSA is essentially applying the scientific method to everyday problems.

Separate training for managers is also necessary because they need to understand and use value-stream maps, PDSA, visual tracking, 6S,[36] and many other tools. ThedaCare managers struggled with lean ideas for months until leaders realized that a lean training course specifically for managers was needed. This course not only taught PDSA, but also prepared managers to mentor others in PDSA.

---

36. 6S stands for sort, straighten, scrub, safety, standardize, sustain—the lean method for workplace organization and visual control. It's an important part of daily improvement where the right layout, supplies, equipment, and information are safely organized and available when needed.

Also, trainers emphasized the potential contradiction between local metrics and ThedaCare's true north metrics, and how value stream maps can interconnect issues—helping managers understand the business case for lean.

ThedaCare's first session attracted 60 people, the second session had 100 attendees, and the next had staff scrounging chairs for 200. They learned to set metrics for their departments consistent with ThedaCare's true north metrics and to manage daily improvement activities while working through their first two PDSAs.

7. Teach a man to fish (or, become a mentor).

There are two basic types of leadership: modern (Sloan) and lean (Toyota). The Sloan style is top-down and autocratic, while lean leaders are teachers and facilitators. Medical and business schools are not churning out Toyota-style leaders, so you will need to create the leaders you want.

Chief executive officers must lead the way to this change by modeling the behavior they want from subordinates. This means being out on the floor where the work takes place, at gemba, with top executives in tow, teaching, listening, and finding barriers to remove for front-line staff. In this way, directors and vice presidents gain first-hand knowledge of lean, see what the new expectations are, and learn to focus their energies on the place where value is created.

CEOs will need to see that bonus structures of top executives are rewritten to reflect lean leadership goals. In the lean world, saving the company money is not rewarded if patient care is undermined in the process. ThedaCare restructured bonuses to reward those who actively participated in improvement work and worked to identify and remove barriers to improvement.

Lean leaders are intimately familiar with work on the front lines. At Autoliv, Inc., a Toyota supplier of auto safety systems, problem-solving is considered a company-wide activity. Once an error or problem is identified, the front-line team member has 15 minutes to find a temporary countermeasure so production can continue safely. If none is found, the supervisor has 15 minutes with the problem before involving a management team. This escalation continues until, if after four hours there is still no countermeasure, the issue lands on the CEO's desk. Imagine if all medication errors were given this type of full-organization scrutiny, with time limits on solving underlying problems that caused the error. Medication errors would fall to zero.

In the perfect lean world ThedaCare is always working toward, every employee is a problem-solver and every executive and manager is a mentor, leading subordinates through a standardized process to solve problems so that they deeply understand what they are trying to accomplish for the organization.

8. Involve suppliers in lean.

Invite suppliers to join lean improvement projects and then set new expectations for how those suppliers interact with your company. In the course of bringing lean to construction suppliers, for instance, ThedaCare employees emphasized mutual cost savings and a long relationship to motivate the suppliers to participate and collaborate in the lean approach.

The key in this work was partnership instead of competition. As part of the 2P process, ThedaCare invited architects and builders to join teams in week-long events focused on care-process redesign. Then, ThedaCare collaborated with its general contractor, Boldt, to create a new delivery model.

Instead of hiring an architect to design a new building and then choosing a builder through competitive bids—a process that typically generates a lot of rework, design changes and cost overruns—ThedaCare now uses an Integrated Lean Project Delivery Core Team. Made up of representatives from ThedaCare, Boldt, and two architectural design firms, the core team has shared responsibility for the design, schedule, and cost of all construction projects.

In fact, the work has resulted in a new, three-way contract between ThedaCare, an architect, and Boldt for each project. The new contract, which can also include a critical supplier, binds all entities together in mutual responsibility.

"We know we're completing projects faster and with less expense," said Albert Park, ThedaCare's Director of Facilities Planning and a licensed architect. "We still don't know how we are doing compared to the wider market. However, we do now have in place a metric to compare our projects to each other, and we are seeing notable improvement."

9. Restructure your organization into product families.

This is a straightforward task in manufacturing where the design and manufacture of different models—for example cars or snow blowers—can be clearly separated into product-family value streams. In healthcare, it means co-locating steps in a process whenever possible to tightly coordinate all the steps of a patient's journey in order to speed value. ThedaCare's experience proves that this is difficult to do in healthcare. Not impossible, but difficult.

For instance, ThedaCare has been working on restructuring several areas to create one musculoskeletal value stream. This involves redesigning patient care in sports medicine, physical therapy, rheumatology, orthopedics, orthopedic surgery, and imaging into a single value stream designed from the customers' perspective. Three years later, improvement teams have moved and streamlined many functions to be more patient-focused, but musculoskeletal, also known as Orthopedics Plus, still does not have a unified financial statement. In addition, there are multiple managers for the various services and there is no single process owner to think about end-to-end improvements.

Over the years, healthcare has added many new treatments, creating many new value streams. These treatments are usually added to the menu in the most cost-effective and convenient way for the healthcare organization, but not always in a way that is convenient or value-creating for the customer.

For instance, as medicine has embraced physical therapy for a wide variety of conditions, hospitals have added gymnasium-type rooms and hired therapists to work in one central location. Essentially, this means that physical therapy is not so much about the patient's condition or convenience as it is about the management of physical therapy. This is not patient-focused care. And yet, when ThedaCare moved some physical therapists out of their central hospital location and into individual clinics, physical therapy revenue dropped by $300,000. That is because Medicare pays less for outpatient-based rehabilitation that it does for inpatient physical therapy.

So, there are roadblocks to creating product families, but this is still important work. Even if it cannot be completed immediately, it will help keep your organization focused on achieving unified, efficient, patient-focused healthcare.

Don't Let Anything Stop You

Once an organization becomes convinced that measurement is necessary, *how* and *what* to measure can become the topic of nagging disagreements and epic turf wars. Do not let that stop the work. This is perhaps the most important piece of advice we can offer from seven years of experience at ThedaCare: trust the improvement process.

Learn everything you can about lean thinking, get all of your top executives on board through hoshin kanri, create an intelligent path, and the infrastructure to support that path. And then keep pushing the work forward.

As top executives in a healthcare organization, we know that there is no substitute for leaders being out on the floor as vocal champions of the work, pushing it constantly forward. If you know that you are saving money and improving patient outcomes—even just a little— then you must continue forward even if you do not yet know the best metrics to portray your success.

Results

While some data are notoriously difficult to capture and publicly share in healthcare, we can report a few big-picture metrics from seven years of lean healthcare work. Further, we believe that any organization that applies the principles and works diligently at improvement can achieve these results.

Access: Same-day appointments are now available at every ThedaCare clinic, every day. Due to lean work, clinical capacity has also expanded and ThedaCare is capable of helping more people.

Price: ThedaCare is consistently the lowest-price overall healthcare provider in the state of Wisconsin. Consumers can visit the Wisconsin Collaborative for Healthcare Quality at www.wchq.org to compare inpatient treatment prices for a variety of diagnoses.

Quality: This is where we have the most trouble compiling and presenting data in a public forum. Individual doctors often have control over what data are released and to whom. Without state or federal mandates, quality reporting is dependent on whim. The Wisconsin Collaborative has won over most of the state's health organizations and reports quality metrics for a number of clinical conditions. ThedaCare is consistently ranked at the top in the state on these measures.

But even here, doctors and surgeons might agree to report only certain types of metrics that may not be entirely useful or clear. At present, we can only offer examples such as ThedaCare's success in reducing the mortality rate for coronary bypass surgery from 4% to near zero, while reducing the cost of that procedure by 22%. In the future, we hope to have more universal—less anecdotal—and relevant quality data.

Staff engagement: On a six-point scale, ThedaCare's mean score on employee opinion surveys rose from 4.485 in 2006 to 5.027 in 2009.

Operating margin: In 2003, ThedaCare's operating margin (profit) was 2.5%. It improved every year since, to 6% in 2009, despite continuing cuts in Medicare reimbursements.

Action Plans for Everyone Else

For those of us working inside the black box that is American health-care, there is plenty of work to do if we are going to save lives and budgets. But what of those people on the outside, debating policy on the state or national level—what is their role? Lean healthcare has three immediate issues.

Healthcare leaders trying to become lean are often stymied by the very policies that outsiders think will help. Instead of more complexity and secrecy, we need sunshine and clarity. In brief, we need:

1. *Mandated consumer reporting for all hospitals, clinics, and care providers detailing quality metrics and cost.* The metrics must be clear and meaningful for patients, such as infection rates and medication errors. This should be built up from existing regional public reporting mechanisms such as the Wisconsin Collaborative for Healthcare Quality. This is a critical need for patients, who do not have free choice when it comes to healthcare providers as long as they lack accurate information. This will be the first step in rewarding quality care throughout the country.

2. *Change government payment criteria to reward quality and lower cost.* Medicare and other public plans should be in the business of stimulating competition between care providers on who can offer the best quality at the best price. At present, they do just the opposite. For example, when ThedaCare found a way to reduce patient stays for given conditions in its Collaborative Care unit while improving outcomes, Medicare's response was to reduce reimbursements by an amount greater than the reduction in stay. ThedaCare was punished for helping patients while saving money.

3. *New insurance strategies working toward universal access should be paid for by taking cost (waste) out of the existing health system, and plans should be administered at the state level.* The federal role should be to set guidelines for quality and access, while state and regional initiatives of key stakeholders banded together in public-private partnerships decide how to redesign the system.

Policymakers will only enact these changes, of course, if patients demand them. Patients—and eventually that includes all of us— need to start demanding clear, easily obtainable, and relevant quality information. Cost comparisons also must be public, because cost affects everyone's ability to access healthcare. We must demand universal access to quality healthcare at lower public costs and stop listening to politicians who say it cannot be done—ThedaCare and many other organizations in the Healthcare Value Leaders Network are now proving that it is imminently possible.

End Note: The Healthcare Value Network

By John Toussaint and Helen Zak

As the ThedaCare medical system continues its journey toward lean healthcare, we have been developing a means for other healthcare organizations to speed their transition from traditional healthcare so the whole industry will be "on the mend." To do this we have formed a partnership between the ThedaCare Center for Healthcare Value (TCHCV) and the Lean Enterprise Institute (LEI), under our joint direction, to launch the Healthcare Value Network (HVN).

The network is a membership organization for healthcare providers in which each provider shares knowledge and findings from its lean journey, including PDSAs and A3s, and hosts joint gemba visits by the other members. Each two-day gemba visit focuses on a specific theme such as hoshin planning, lean leadership, or yokoten. The host and the attendees share current knowledge about the subject and build relationships for continuing knowledge exchanges.

The network also utilizes a private collaboration site through the Healthcare Value Network website where the members share videos, examples of standard work, PDSAs, A3s, and other knowledge useful for transformation. It also allows for affinty groups to share knowledge with each other. These materials are supplemented by learning modules, prepared by the HVN staff, for use by the members.

Each member of the network may participate in a lean assessment, developed in cooperation with the Shingo Prize organization at Utah State University, to determine where the organization is on its lean journey. The assessment is then used to understand and remedy gaps in knowledge and performance.

The premise of the network is that the participating organizations will be able to progress faster through collaboration than they would be able to alone and the initial results have been very encouraging. However, the context in which healthcare is provided is also critical, in particular the way healthcare providers are reimbursed by governments and insurers and the way that healthcare outcomes are reported to funding sources and the public. These issues are being addressed by the ThedaCare Center for Healthcare Value through research and frequent interaction with legislators, policymakers in governments, and other policy research organizations. At the same time, there is a need to spread awareness that lean principles, initially developed in manufacturing industries, are highly effective in healthcare. Refining the principles of lean thinking and publicizing their relevance to healthcare has been a focus of the Lean Enterprise Institute for more than a decade. Together, we believe that TCHCV, LEI, and HVN can play a powerful role in raising consciousness about what is possible and can continually create and then share knowledge about the path to lean transformation.

We hope that any healthcare provider committed to fundamentally changing its approach to service delivery will consider joining the Healthcare Value Network. For more information and to apply for membership, please visit *createvalue.org/delivery/hvn*

For more information about the ThedaCare Center for Healthcare Value, visit *createvalue.org*

For more information about the Lean Enterprise Institute, visit *lean.org*

Acknowledgments

In this work, we have been helped by many to understand our journey and the challenges we faced along the way. We will not be able to name them all here, but some do stand out for specific acknowledgment.

Specific thanks to Jamie Dunham, Dr. Mark Hallett, Kathryn Correia, Dr. Joyce Bauer, Bill Boyd, Richard Berry, Lee Parker, Cindy Krueger, Myrtle Bellis and others who had the courage to tell us the truth about their experiences—the good, the bad, and the ugly—and allow their names to stand next to their stories. They are truly living our value of candor with respect.

Also, special thanks to Jacci Huss, Kimberly Zwiers, Peggy Bree, Sally Podoski, Dan Collins and countless others from inside ThedaCare who helped us track down data and people to bring this story to life.

George Koenigsaecker, our most important mentor, was there through thick and thin to coach, cajole, and critically evaluate the work. Along with the experts from Simpler Consulting, George taught us the core components of lean while we taught him the world of healthcare.

Don Berwick and Maureen Bisognano at the Institute for Healthcare Improvement started us on the continuous-improvement journey almost 20 years ago and have never stopped encouraging innovation and new ways to improve patient care.

Without Dan Ariens' willingness to share his own experience with lean manufacturing, we would not have learned the fundamental lean principles. Ariens—the company and its executives—is one of the major reasons ThedaCare has been successful.

We also owe a debt to ThedaCare's board and board chairs including John Nussbaum, former CEO of Plexus, Paul Karch of the legal firm Godfrey and Kahn, and Walter Rugland, former COO of Thrivent. These leaders made us believe in ourselves in the worst of times.

Thank you to Dean Gruner, MD, CEO of ThedaCare; Jeff Thompson, MD, CEO of Gundersen Lutheran in Lacrosse, WI; Chris Queram, CEO of the Wisconsin Collaborative for Healthcare Quality; Don Logan, MD, former chief medical officer of Dean Health System; George Kerwin, CEO of Bellin Health; Carl Westbrook, MD, former CEO of Marshfield Clinic; and Bud Chumbley, MD, former president of ProHealth Care Medical Associates; all of whom are dedicated to transparency in medical outcomes reporting and helped John establish the Wisconsin Collaborative for Healthcare Quality.

A special thanks to Helen Zak and Mark Graban, the Lean Enterprise Institute's experts on healthcare, for their support throughout the development process and to Jane Bulnes-Fowles and Thomas Skehan for their help in producing this book. And special, special thanks to Emily Adams for helping us clearly articulate our experience on the printed page and precisely capture ThedaCare's remarkable story.

We gratefully acknowledge those we hold close and dear: our spouses, family members, colleagues, and friends. They have had to endure our newfound "expertise" about lean, as we have ranted about the waste we now seem to find everywhere we go, including the ice cream parlor, the grocery store, the school system, and even our places of worship. Thank you for tenaciously reminding us that life is about more than mere efficiency, but also about the very human nature of the journey that we are all on.

Appendix

Figure 1: Collaborative Care Results

Collaborative Care Results to Date			
Measure	**Pre-collaborative care (2006)**	**End of 2007**	
Defect-free Admission Medication Reconciliation	**1.05 defects** per chart	**0.01 defects** per chart (-99% vs. 2006)	
Quality Bundle Compliance	**38% Pneumonia** (2005 baseline) No baseline for CHF	**100% Pneumonia** **92.5% CHF**	
Patient Satisfaction	**68%** rated as top box	**87%** (+30% vs. 2006)	
Length of Stay*	**3.71 days**	**2.96 days** (-20% vs. 2006)	
Case Mix Index* Used top 16 DRGs that match across cc and non-cc	**1.08**	**1.12**	
Average Cost Per Case* (using Medicare RCC)	**$5,669** fully loaded	**$4,467** fully loaded (-21% s. 2006)	

*

End of 2008	2009	Compared to non-collaborative care
0 defects	0 defects	1.25 defects per chart without RPh
95% Pneumonia 85% CHF	95% Pneumonia 92% CHF	83% Pneumonia (all or none bundle score) 90% CHF (all or none bundle score)
90%	4.5 on a scale of 5 (revised tool in Sept. 2008)	Not captured for other units
3.16 days	3.01 days	3.19 days
1.11	1.13	1.37
$5,849	$5,567 fully loaded	$7,775

*Financial Indicators represent a subset of the patients to demonstrate impact of the delivery model. Excluded from both baseline and pilot are: observation patients, ICU patients, and LOS >15 days. Pilot numbers includes: Admits from ED to Unit, or direct admits to unit. 2006 is updated baseline.

Figure 2: Initial STEMI Value-Stream Map 2005

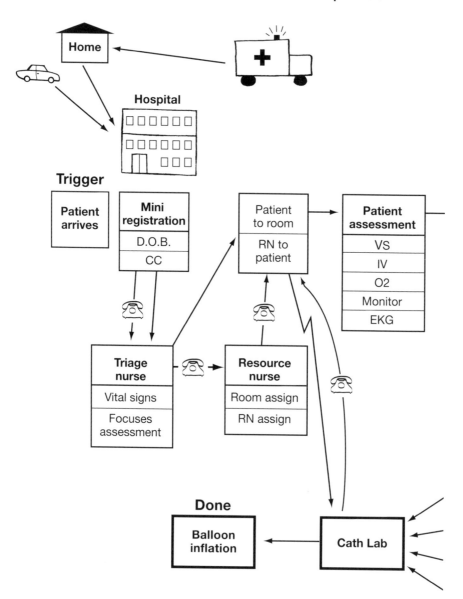

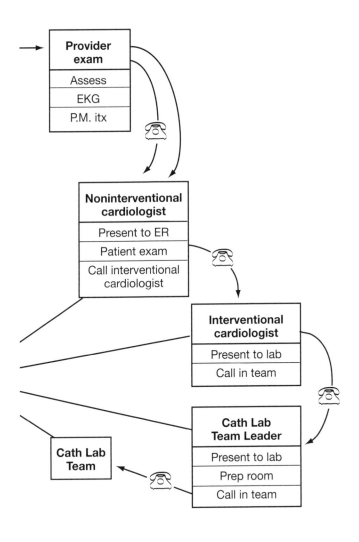

Figure 3: Improved STEMI Value-Stream Map 2010

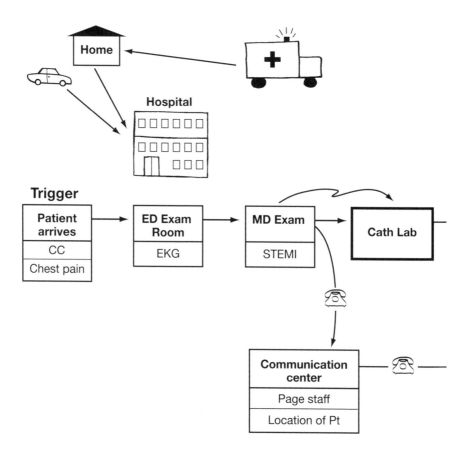

Done

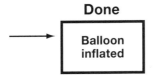

Balloon
inflated

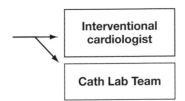

Interventional
cardiologist

Cath Lab Team

Figure 4: Code Stroke Process Flow

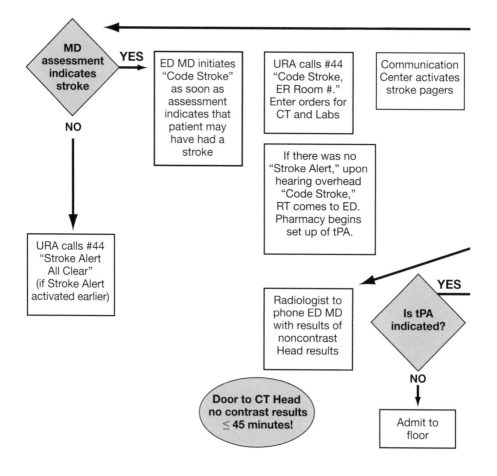

| URA calls on 44 line "Stroke Alert, ETA/Room #" | Patient arrives in ED via EMS. Verbal report from EMS to ED. | MD/RN assessment | Start Code Stroke Flow Sheet |

| Upon hearing overhead "Stroke Alert," RT comes to ED. Pharmacy begins set up of tPA. | Patient arrives in ED via walk in. |

AA registers patient based on EMS report

| Patient taken to CT | RN calls pharmacy with weight and allergies while patient in CT. Pharmacy will calculate tPA dosage. (Will not mix yet.) | Neurology calls ED and talks to ER MD | Continue Stroke Flow Sheet – Priority 2 or 3 (if ordered) |

Door to CT ≤ 25 minutes!

| ED faxes tPA order and calls pharmacy to indicate order has been faxed | Pharmacy mixes tPA | Pharmacy hand delivers tPA to patient room | tPa administered to patient |

Door to start tPA ≤ 60 minutes!

On the Mend

Figure 5: Detail of Visual Matrix Diagram Used in Hoshin Kanri

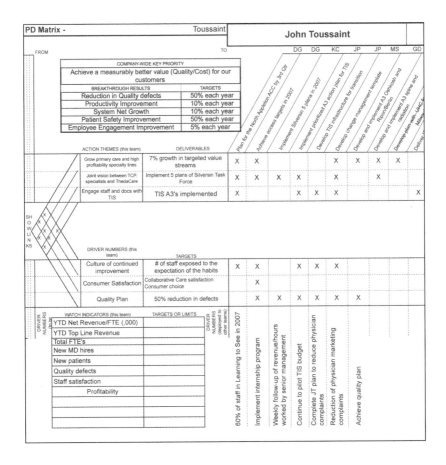

Figure 6: PDSA A3 Template

Title:	Fresh Eyes:
Owner:	Team:
PDSA:	
Coach:	

PLAN

Background/Current conditions

Problem statement

Goals/Targets

Stakeholder Signatures:

Subject Expert(s):	Start Date:
	Revision Date:
	Revision Number:

PLAN	**Analysis/Root cause**	
DO	**Countermeasures to root causes**	
STUDY	**Study (planned vs. actual results)**	
ACT/ADJUST	**Act/Adjust**	

Figure 7: Results of the ThedaCare Employee Satisfaction Survey 2004–2008

This annual survey is on a six-point scale.

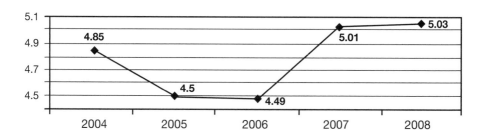

Figure 8: Standard Work for Supervisors

AMC CVS Day Supervisor Standard Work

Last updated	Owner	**Julie RN BSN**	Performed by **Supervisor**	Work In Process **1**
Takt time	Revised by		Rev. Number	
	Trigger	**0800**	Done	

Time	Major Steps	Details	a	Reasons (why)
0800–0815	Assess Unit Needs	Gemba with Manager, VP, Clinical Lead Update stat sheet, Scorecard, Communication Board		
0815–0830		Discuss project work with Manager and VP		
0830–0900	Stat sheet	Attend Bed Meeting		
0900–1200	Go to Gemba	Review communcation with Lead as to what needs to be passed on in a huddle New/updated standard work Incident report follow-up Teach in the work Model/coach/correct Standard Work Round on Unit Complete meeting agendas Make additions to Bypass Complete e-mails		
1200–1230	Assess 14:00 staffing	Meet with Clinical Lead to assess staffing needs for the PM shift		
1230–1600	Work time	Lunch Office/project work E-mail/phone messages Additional time on the Gemba Teach in the work Model/coach/audit and correct Standard Work		
1600–1630	Assess 18:00 staffing	Attend meeting with Lead/C- Spa		

Figure 9: Standard Work for Managers

Manager Morning Standard Work		
Last updated **10/15/09**	Owner	**Kim**
	Revised by	**Patsy**
Takt time **2 hours**	Trigger	**0800 each morning**

	Major Steps	Details (if applicable)
1	Stat sheet	Update stat sheet with Supervisor Remove barriers—escalate when appropriate
2	Defect Huddle	(See huddle SW) • Identify defects • Create assignments • Establish daily priorities with the team • Establish the discipline of daily follow through as a team.
3	Go to the Gemba	**Understand the work of the day** **Tone should be uplifting and supportive** • Stand in the circle and observe the flow, seek to understand. Identify defects. Develop a plan to share with the team. • Bring supervisor at least weekly to stand in the circle with you. Learn to see together. Focus on Flow. • Team Building—recognize staff for good work **Communication** • Plan a intentional conversation with individual staff that shows you support them and their work • Provide positive reinforcement and/or constructive feedback **Coaching/Mentoring** • Reinforce link between work staff are doing to unit goals • Encourage them to problem-solve defects with the team and bring forth potential top contributors and solutions approaches • Model PDSA thinking • Support continuous learning • Model/coach/correct Standard Work • Teach in the work **Audit: Will need a process to audit priority SW** • Everyday audit a piece of SW and twice a week do it with your supervisor • Identify actual errors/defects • Use in the moment teaching **Problem-Solving: Managing improvement capacity and flow of problem-solving** • Apply TIS tools • Follow up with lead to problem-solve • Find and eliminate the root cause • If safety issue identified, identify immediate containment plan and communicate **Visibility and access to team and physicians**

Performed by	**Manager**	Work In Process
Rev. Number	**2**	
Done		

Reasons (why)

To develop and coach the supervisor. To provide high-level understandings of work flow to VP and escalate defects for additional support.

To review yesterday's defects and identify opportunities for improvement on a daily basis. Support, teach, and develop PDSA thinking with the team. Used to determine work of day a nd proactively assess issues. Barrier removal and escalation.

To understand your business. To understand and improve the flow of your unit. To maintain and improve standards, and address any variation. Also, to develop our people by teaching to standard and modeling problem-solving (PDSA).

Figure 10: Standard Work Sample Schedule (Furlan)

November 2009				
16 Monday	**17 Tuesday**	**18 Wednesday**	**19 Thursday**	**20 Friday**
Early				
7:00 AM				
8:00 AM (8:00 – 10:00 AM) **NO MEETING ZONE** TC Heritage	(8:00 – 10:00 AM) **NO MEETING ZONE** TC Admin Conf Rm	(8:00 – 12:00 PM) HLT (Operations) (location changed)	(8:00 – 10:00 AM) **NO MEETING ZONE** TC Heritage	(8:00 – 9:00 AM) Report Out Bordini Center
9:00 AM				(9:30 – 10:30 AM) BPS Friday Reflection
10:00 AM (10:00 – 11:00 AM) Do Not Schedule	(10:00 AM – 12:30 PM) Do Not Schedule		(10:00 AM – 12:30 PM) Do Not Schedule	(10:30 – 11:30 AM) Do Not Schedule
11:00 AM (11:00 – 11:30 AM) Travel (11:30 AM – 12:30 PM) HOF Core Team Meeting				(11:30 AM – 12:15 PM) Rich Maxwell
12:00 PM (12:30 – 1:00 PM) Review plan for Dec. Leadership Preapation Project	(12:30 – 2:00 PM) **DO NOT MOVE** Conf Call w/Kathryn & Matt	(12:00 – 1:30 PM) Do Not Schedule	(12:30 – 2:30 PM) Employee Safety PDSA Weekly Mtg. (time expanded) TC Heritage (cg)	(12:15 – 1:00 PM) Do Not Schedule
1:00 PM (1:00 – 4:00 PM) Strategy Deployment		(1:30 – 2:30 PM) Meeting w/Mia, Kathryn & Matt (every other month) @ Corp Shores		(1:00 – 2:00 PM) Weekly 1:1 Jodi/Matt
2:00 PM	(2:00 – 4:00 PM) Do Not Schedule	(2:30 – 3:30 PM) Do Not Schedule	(2:30 – 4:30 PM) Hospital Managers' Meeting	(2:00 – 4:00 PM) Oshkosh Strategy X 8,7555
3:00 PM		(3:30 – 3:45 PM) Capital Documents for November Board Packet		
4:00 PM	(4:00 – 4:30 PM) Development Plans	(4:00 – 4:30 PM) Customer Service		
5:00 PM				
Late				

Figure 11: Five Stages of Change

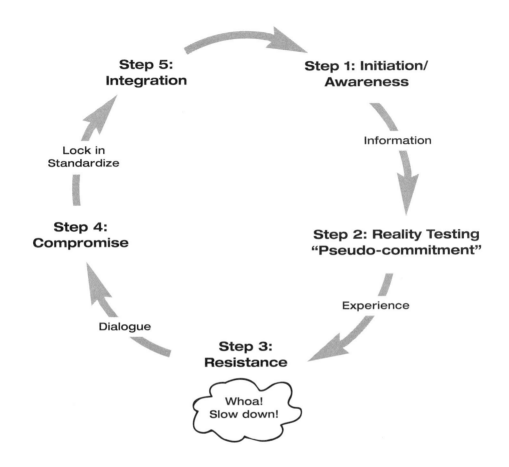

Figure 12: Employee Engagement Results

	Total (N=3,583)	Number of RIEs				F	P
		0 (N=2,370)	1 (N=726)	2–5 (N=425)	6 or more (N=62)		
1) My manager shows appreciation for the work I do.	2.97	2.93	2.96	3.10	3.55	18.26	0.0
2) People are encouraged to balance their work and personal life.	2.86	2.85	2.83	2.96	3.15	7.23	0.0
3) I would recommend this organization to a friend as a good place to work.	3.15	3.13	3.11	3.28	3.64	19.13	0.0
4) Mangement has kept promises made to us.	2.79	2.76	2.77	2.91	3.30	15.55	0.0
5) My manager or someone at work seems to care about me as a person.	3.13	3.09	3.14	3.24	3.57	16.80	0.0
6) I am satisfied with my job security.	2.97	2.95	2.95	3.08	3.33	10.48	0.0
7) My manager provides me with sufficient opportunities to improve myself.	2.92	2.89	2.90	3.06	3.45	20.85	0.0
8) At work, my opinions seem to count.	2.78	2.73	2.79	2.97	3.52	32.77	0.0
9) People here are willing to give extra to get the job done.	3.06	3.05	3.03	3.09	3.50	10.51	0.0
10) Overall, I think this is a great place to work.	3.15	3.13	3.14	3.24	3.61	17.16	0.0

Nancy Gurnee "Employee Satisfaction and Lean Production Methods in Healthcare Organization" (master's thesis) University of Wisconsin 2006, p. 22.

Figure 13: True North Metrics

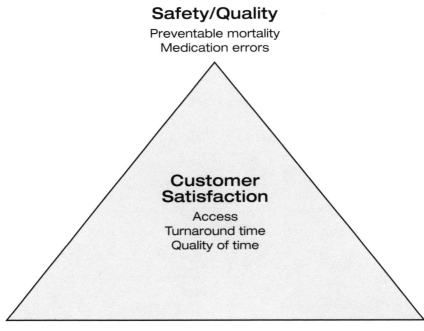

True North Metrics

Safety/Quality
Preventable mortality
Medication errors

**Customer
Satisfaction**

Access
Turnaround time
Quality of time

People
OSHA Recordable injuries
HAT Scores

Financial
Stewardship
Operating margin
Productivity

Index